D0050651

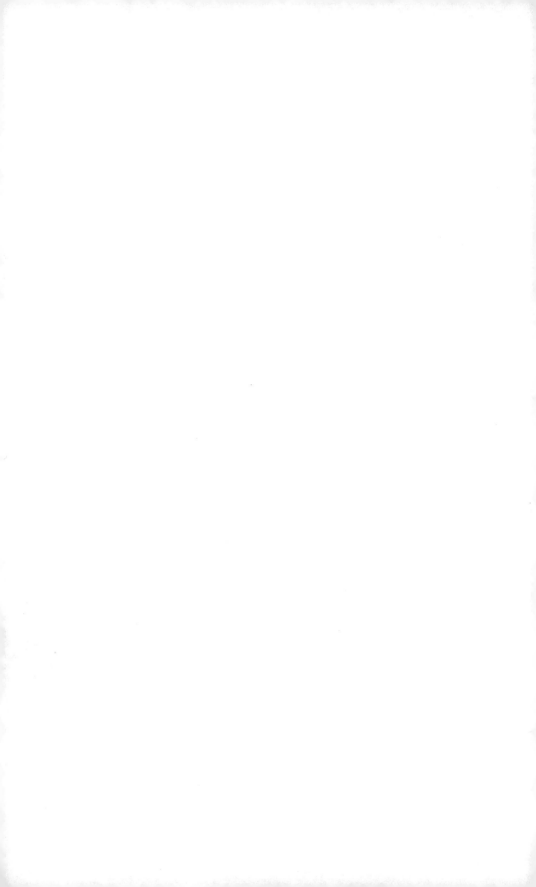

The
Anticancer
Diet

The Anticancer Diet

Reduce Cancer Risk Through the Foods You Eat

....

David Khayat, MD

WITH COLLABORATION FROM

Nathalie Hutter-Lardeau
and France Carp

W. W. NORTON & COMPANY

NEW YORK • LONDON

No book can replace the diagnostic expertise and medical advice of a trusted physician. Please consult with your doctor if you are experiencing pain or other symptons of illness, or if you have been diagnosed with any medical condition that requires ongoing care.

Translated by Morag Jordan

Copyright © 2010 by Odile Jacob
Translation copyright © 2015 by W. W. Norton & Company, Inc.

Originally published in French as LE VRAI REGIME ANTICANCER

For information about permission to reproduce selections from this book, write to Permissions, W. W. Norton & Company, Inc., 500 Fifth Avenue, New York, NY 10110

For information about special discounts for bulk purchases, please contact W. W. Norton Special Sales at specialsales@wwnorton.com or 800-233-4830

Manufacturing by Courier Westford
Production manager: Anna Oler

Library of Congress Cataloging-in-Publication Data

Khayat, David.
[Vrai régime anticancer. English]
The anticancer diet : reduce cancer risk through the foods you eat / David Khayat, M.D. ; with collaboration from Nathalie Hutter-Lardeau and France Carp.
pages cm
Includes bibliographical references and index.
ISBN 978-0-393-08893-9 (hardcover)
1. Cancer—Diet therapy. 2. Cancer—Nutritional aspects. 3. Cancer—Prevention—Nutritional aspects. I. Hutter-Lardeau, Nathalie. II. Carp, France. III. Title.
RC271.D52K5313 2015
616.99'40654—dc23
2015000661

W. W. Norton & Company, Inc.
500 Fifth Avenue, New York, N.Y. 10110
www.wwnorton.com

W. W. Norton & Company Ltd.
Castle House, 75/76 Wells Street, London W1T 3QT

1 2 3 4 5 6 7 8 9 0

To my mother and father,
who by giving me food gave me so much love.

To my wife and to my darling girls,
*our family meals
were such fun when we
were all together!
I miss them.*

My thanks to the people who have
helped me write this book:
to Virginie Baffet,
for being so efficient,
to the whole wonderful team at
Atlantic Santé,
and to my friend Roger Mouawad,
always there when I need him.

Contents

Preface

....

At the time I wrote this book in French, it was exactly thirty years since I had started my professional battle against cancer.

On September 1, 1980, I arrived in the Medical Oncology Department at the Pitié-Salpétrière Hospital in central Paris.

Thirty years!

I started as an intern at the Paris Public Hospitals, then became an assistant professor, and, a little later, earned my doctorate in medicine. After carrying out research in Israel and then in New York, I earned a second doctorate in human biology.

I was appointed professor of oncology at the Pierre-et-Marie-Curie University in Paris and then given the same appointment as an adjunct professor at the University of Texas at the MD Anderson Cancer Center. Twenty years ago, I became head of the Medical Oncology Department at the Pitié-Salpétrière Hospital. At the request of then French president Jacques Chirac, from 2002 to 2006 I was responsible for the national cancer plan for France.

And throughout all these years, whatever my title, position, or responsibility, the central thread in my life has always been to treat and look after cancer patients.

For over thirty years I've been striving to gain a better understanding of cancer, to fight it better, and to get the better of it more often. I've never given up trying, through endless research, through exchanges with my colleagues (who are the most eminent scientists across the world), through reading absolutely everything available on the subject, and by sounding out ideas and theories with the greatest minds in the field of cancer.

I've waged this battle alongside thousands of patients, developing a closeness to them that was often akin to true friendship.

I've often helped them toward recovery; however, too often, I've seen them die as well.

I've tried by every means possible to prevent cancer from spreading inside their bodies; at times this involved using procedures so innovative that they seemed totally crazy.

In close combat, with patient after patient, confronting all these countless, mysterious cancers, one after the other—a little like a soldier fighting with only a knife for a weapon—I've attempted to steer my patients to victory, to recovery.

These battles have been so hard, and my patients' suffering has been so great. At every moment throughout my life, sorrow and frustration have been my companions.

With the plan that I suggested to President Chirac, I tried to score some points back from this disease, no longer by fighting for individual patients case by case, but by setting up national strategies to fight cancer: developing screening programs and early diagnostic tests; ensuring that wherever patients were in France, they could all benefit from the very latest treatment; and stimulating scientific research and the development of new tools that would mean better care for all these patients.

However, tragically we are forced to admit that victory still eludes us. At this stage in my life, it seems clear that a very long time ago something should have been done or, in any case, been developed further —and that is prevention.

That is why I wanted to write this book and set down my thirty years of experience and thoughts. I wanted to impart all my knowledge so that it can be shared with as many people as possible, so that together we can speak about hope and tell ourselves that thanks to all the work done, our children will perhaps one day live in a world that is rid of the threat of this "nasty disease" once and for all!

Unlike the people who want to draw up rules based on their own particular, personal experience of cancer, rules that they would like to impose on everyone else, without even exercising the caution of qualifiers such as "might," "possibly," and so on, as befits any proper researcher, this book is the sum of my over thirty years of research into cancer, both in laboratories and at patients' bedsides, in France and in the United States. Its legitimacy is beyond dispute, especially as it's the result of a successful collaboration between a cancer specialist and a preeminent nutritionist.

DAVID KHAYAT
April 2010

The
Anticancer
Diet

Introduction

···

Breast cancer is far less common in Japanese women than in American women. Why is this so?

An even more surprising question is, why is it that when Japanese women emigrate to the United States, from the second generation onward, they're at as much risk of developing breast cancer as American women?

Has the genetic makeup of these Japanese women suddenly changed? Of course not, nothing of the sort! They still look just like Japanese women, and in their outward appearance nothing has changed.

Have they been subjected to some sort of carcinogenic process? Is there really so much more pollution in American cities than in Tokyo or Osaka? Definitely not. Quite obviously neither is true!

Then how do we explain this phenomenon? What is happening to these women that within scarcely two generations, a risk so significant, so specific, and so life-threatening can be modified to this extent?

In actual fact, only one thing has happened, and it demonstrates vividly what this book is all about.

Within two generations, these women have changed their habits, and in particular their eating habits. Unfortunately for them, they have adopted the diet of American women, what we term the "Westernization" of food. This second generation of women eats less fish, rice, fruit, and vegetables and includes in its daily diet more meat, fat in all its various guises, as well as sweet, sugary foods. They tend to become plumper and drink more sugary soft drinks, thereby boosting their daily calorie intake. By doing all these things, and without our being able to explain it definitively, they've dramatically increased their likelihood of developing a malignant breast tumor.

When we look at the geographical spread for the risk of cancer, by the type of cancer or by country, we cannot help but be struck by the incredible differences we often see. There is far more bowel (colon) cancer in Australia and New Zealand than in France or Italy. Stomach cancer is far less common in Germany than in Japan or Uganda. The risk of getting breast cancer is strikingly greater in England than in Greece. Skin cancer is far more common in Israel than in Ireland.

And we could carry on listing these examples ad infinitum!

So how do we explain these statistics? There are, of course, genetic differences between the populations in these different countries. In addition, certain infectious agents that cause more contamination in one place than in another, and are potentially carcinogenic, may also account for a particular difference in a particular place.

However, when reading the studies that attempt to throw light on these mysteries, what we call "epidemiological" studies, to which we'll return later, we cannot help but reach the conclusion that our eating habits have played a role in what's happening with cancer. In isolation or in combination with other risk factors, to a significant or at times quite marginal and barely detectable extent, it's our eating habits that are responsible for all these differences.

The truth is that our eating habits, in the broadest sense, are in fact responsible for many of the cancers we get!

Chapter 1

······················

Cancer

CHOOSING PREVENTION

··

O ur eating habits are responsible for many cancers. No doubt this would be of no significance if over the years cancer had not become for the whole of humanity the terrible scourge that it is now. In the Western world, nearly one in two men is or will be affected by cancer, and more than one in three women. In 2000, there were ten million new cases of cancer worldwide, resulting in six million deaths per year. For 2020, only a few years away, the World Health Organization (WHO) forecasts twenty million new cases and ten million deaths.[1]

Not only does cancer kill more people across the world than AIDS, but it kills more people than AIDS and tuberculosis and malaria combined.[2] In the United States, although AIDS unfortunately still kills around 9,400 people each year, cancer kills 585,000 American citizens annually.

Contrary to what many think, cancer is the leading cause of mortality in adults, and this is true for poor countries too.[3, 4]

In 2010, in the United States, almost five women died every hour from breast cancer. In Europe, a third of deaths are caused by cancer. In France, since 2009, cancer has become the main cause of death.

And let's stop thinking that "it's quite normal to die of cancer as cancer kills old people and we all have to die one day!" What nonsense!

TABLE 1-1

**ESTIMATED NUMBER OF NEW CANCER CASES AND DEATHS BY SEX
FOR SELECTED SITES, UNITED STATES, 2014, ACCORDING TO THE
AMERICAN CANCER SOCIETY[5]**

Sites	MALE		FEMALE	
	New cases	Deaths	New cases	Deaths
Oral and cavity pharynx	30,220	5,730	12,220	2,660
Esophagus	18,170	12,450	3,510	3,000
Stomach	13,730	6,720	8,490	4,270
Colon, rectum*	71,830	26,270	65,000	24,040
Liver and intrahepatic bile duct	24,600	15,870	8,590	7,130
Pancreas	23,530	20,170	2,890	9,420
Larynx	10,000	2,870	2,630	740
Lung and bronchus	116,000	86,930	108,210	72,330
Skin: Melanoma	43,890	6,470	32,210	3,240
Breast	2,360	430	232,670	40,000
Uterine cervix	—	—	12,360	4,020
Uterine corpus	—	—	52,630	8,590
Ovary	—	—	21,980	14,270
Prostate	233,000	29,480	—	—
Testis	8,820	380	—	—
Urinary bladder	56,390	11,170	18,300	4,410
Kidney and renal pelvis	39,140	8,900	24,780	4,960
Brain and other nervous system	12,820	8,090	10,560	6,230
Thyroid	15,190	830	47,790	1,060
Lymphoma	43,340	11,140	36,650	9,030
Myeloma	13,500	6,110	10,550	4,980
Leukemia	30,100	14,040	22,280	10,050
All sites[†]	1,665,540	299,200	739,940	270,290

Note: All leukemias are grouped together.
* Deaths are combined.
[†] Including sites not listed in above table.

In the United States, cancer is the leading cause of premature mortality in men aged forty-five to sixty-four. Tobacco alone is accountable for around 5.1 million years of potential life lost in people younger than seventy-five in the United States.

(Note that this covers all deaths from tobacco use, including cardiovascular disease.)[6, 7]

IT WOULD HAVE BEEN WONDERFUL if all those years had been lived. And the loss of people is also a loss to economic growth. If the direct cost of treating cancer in the United States amounts to around $103 billion, the indirect cost due to these premature deaths adds a further $161 billion.

Overall, cancer costs the United States around $264 billion each year, an enormous sum![8]

The WHO has made clear that the number of cancers is doubling every twenty years.

So where are we heading? How can we deal with such a terrible loss of all these men and women still in the prime of life? Where will we

TABLE 1-2

INCIDENCE OF CANCER IN 2008 AND ESTIMATES FOR 2030 (IN MILLIONS)[9]

Region	Number of cases in 2008	Estimate of the number of cases in 2030 (without any change in the incidence rate)	Estimate of the number of cases in 2030 (with an annual 1% increase in the incidence rate)
Africa	0.7	1.2	1.6
Europe	3.4	4.1	5.5
Mediterranean Region	0.5	0.9	1.2
North America	2.6	4.8	6.4
Southeast Asia	1.6	2.8	3.7
Western Pacific	3.7	6.1	8.1
Worldwide	12.4	20	26.4

find the money to fund the ever-growing cost of treating their illness? If we do nothing to change the factors determining this situation, plainly we're heading toward disaster.

HOW CAN WE LESSEN OUR RISK OF CANCER?

So what can we do? The answer is simple: other than quickly coming up with a miracle treatment that will turn cancer into nothing more threatening than a common cold, we have no other alternative than to commit ourselves to fighting cancer with unwavering determination in the best, least costly, and yet, at the same time, most effective way—which is to prevent it.

Preventing cancer, preventing it from even developing, is quite logically still the most realistic and most acceptable strategy we can adopt as we try to eradicate this dreadful scourge.

But how do we do this? Faced with a monster that is so fearsome, so voracious for death-inducing growth, so complex and multifaceted, how can we imagine any processes, mechanisms, or attitudes that could stop a malignant tumor from developing?

As its French name *maligne* makes clear, and it wasn't chosen by chance, this disease is malignant, cunning, and insidious!

Cancer doesn't allow us easy access to weapons that can potentially deal with it. And perhaps most importantly, it is best to treat it, not once it has become all too apparent, but when it's still in its earliest stages, lurking away in a hidden corner of the body of a person who still doesn't feel even slightly unwell. When it's in the breast or the prostate, quietly waiting to be fed, so it can grow and spread. When prevention could still avert the disease, all the stressful treatments required—such as surgery, radiotherapy, and chemotherapy—and sometimes death.

For us to be able to give careful thought to these prevention strategies, which are so important and yet so difficult to imagine, we'll need to briefly review what we know about what "gives us cancer."

Later on in this book, we'll take a much closer look at a cancerous cell, and together we'll attempt to understand how it turns into such a formidable enemy. We'll do this, not with the aim of being able to impart complex, academic knowledge gained from the millions of scientific articles published annually. No, we'll do it in an extremely simplified way to show how a food that we ingest—for example, an orange or a steak—can disrupt a mechanism that regulates life in one of our cells, and transform it into a cancerous cell, or conversely, how a food is able to protect the cell.

At this stage in our undertaking, we'll simply examine the causes—in medical language, the etiologies—of our cancers to see how, by changing a particular parameter, we might be able to prevent the cancer from spreading.

Tobacco is the main cause of cancer

The causes of cancers are extremely varied, as are indeed the types of cancers that exist. However, one thing is sure, holding true throughout the world: by far, the primary cause of cancer is tobacco, in whatever form it is taken and however it is used. Globally, tobacco accounts for 25–30% of all cancers.[10]

Tobacco alone causes a third of cancers.

Whether smoked or chewed, in cigarettes or a pipe, low-tobacco cigarettes or not, filtered or unfiltered, tobacco causes cancer. It gives us cancer of our lips, mouth, larynx, bronchi, lungs, esophagus, stomach, pancreas, kidneys, bladder, and so on. While in proportions that vary from one cancer to the next, it accounts for up to 70% of lung and throat cancer cases. Whether working alone or alongside other carcinogenic factors—we'll come back to this—tobacco is a fearsome agent in the carcinogenesis process in cells. Tobacco products that get into our bodies as we inhale or swallow them naturally find their way inside our most fragile cells. By reacting chemically with our DNA (that is, with our genes imprinted into our chromosomes), tobacco causes a whole series of mutations, which in turn lead to cells becoming malignant and the onset of cancer.

And you should be aware that this holds equally true for products

TABLE 1-3

TOBACCO-RELATED CANCERS[11]

Site of the cancer	Percentage of cancers due to smoking	
	Men	Women
Oral cavity	63	17
Pharynx	76	44
Esophagus	51	34
Stomach	31	14
Liver	38	17
Pancreas	25	17
Larynx	76	65
Lung	83	69
Kidney	26	12
Bladder	53	39
Cervix	—	23

Note: The data pertain to France; there are no comparable data available for the United States.

made from other types of plants that some people choose to smoke, such as marijuana.

That some cigarettes contain less tobacco than others does nothing to lessen their risk. The only thing it does is make the smoker inhale their puffs of tobacco more deeply. Cancers will then develop more around the lungs, which is precisely what we observe.[12, 13]

Across the world, the number of deaths due to tobacco is permanently on the increase and is going to pose some very serious problems, especially in China, where over 2 billion of the 5.5 billion cigarettes produced annually are smoked.

If you are a smoker, you should not fool yourself by trying to eat "organic" foods or follow some sort of life-saving diet. Compared with the direct role tobacco plays in the origin of most cancers and its incredible impact, any attempt at prevention you carry out while still continuing to smoke will count for absolutely nothing, and thinking that you're doing some good is nothing but an illusion!

So the first rule we'll lay down in our "true anticancer diet" is DON'T SMOKE.

Nowadays, there are centers in just about every hospital that give advice on quitting smoking. For those who need them, nicotine substitutes can be very useful. Anyone who wants to avoid cancer and who smokes can start by doing a very simple thing: give up smoking!

Better still—never start smoking in the first place! This advice is directed most especially to young people, our children.

You know now that wherever you live in the world, smoking is the primary cause of cancer, responsible for a third of cancers. So what causes the remaining 70%?

The carcinogenic effect of hormones

Another third of cancers is due to the effect that natural or artificial hormones (as in replacement therapies for menopause) have on specific organs that are sensitive to them. This is true for female hormones, estrogens, and breast cancer and cancer of the womb, and for the male hormone, testosterone, and prostate cancer.

In the United States, the most common of these cancers are breast cancer in women and prostate cancer in men, resulting in approximately 40,000 and 32,000 deaths each year, respectively.

Can we do anything to help prevent them? Our answer is both yes and no!

You should know that for a woman the risk is much greater if:

- Her mother or sister had breast cancer.
- She went through puberty early.
- Her first pregnancy was late.
- She's had few children.
- She didn't breastfeed.
- Her menopause was late.
- If at menopause, she used hormone replacement therapy (HRT) over a long period.

As we can immediately see, apart from not taking HRT when menopause is normal, there's little we can do. We can't choose at what age we go through puberty or menopause. We can't influence the illnesses that our parents might have developed. We can't compel women to have more children and have them earlier on! So, a priori, the answer to the question "Can we prevent these cancers by acting on our hormones?" is no. However, as we'll see later, we do have enough scientific data today to nonetheless remain hopeful and to answer this question by saying yes, to some extent it is possible, if we're careful about what we eat. Hormonal status is related inevitably to what we eat. And the same goes for prostate cancer in men.

So we have dealt with 60% of cancers, half due to tobacco and half to our hormones. Now we just have to explain the remaining 40%.

Infectious agents and environmental causes of cancers

For one-half (20%) of the remaining cases of all cancers, the causes come down to a whole array of etiological factors, on the one hand, and will be subject to great variability from one place to another across the world, on the other.

Some cancers result from the carcinogenic action of an infectious agent. Few people are aware of this, but many cancers are directly connected to an infection in an organ from specific bacteria or viruses.

This is true of cancers of the cervix, liver, stomach, mouth, penis, anus, bladder, and lymph glands. In fact, the better we get at detecting the presence of viruses in tumors, the more new cancers we discover connected to them.

Although it has been long known that liver cancers are caused by the hepatitis virus, it was only at the end of 2006 that we discovered that the majority of cancers of the mouth are also caused by a virus, in this case human papillomavirus (HPV), the same virus that causes cervical cancer and that can be caught from having oral sex.

The theory that a virus or, at any rate, an infection (caused by bacteria, virus, parasite, etc.) is responsible for some cancers is becoming increasingly popular again among cancer specialists. A certain number of these infectious carcinogenic agents will contaminate us through what we eat and, in particular, through what we drink. We'll return later to this link between our diet and cancer.

I wouldn't be surprised if, in years to come, the proportion of cancers caused by infectious agents were to rise from the 5% we know today to reach 20% or 30%.

Pollution is another cause of cancer and accounts for nearly 5%. It encompasses agricultural pollutants, which explain the leukemias and some other cancers that are very common among agricultural workers. Urban consumers come across the pollutants in fruits and vegetables.

We come into contact with pollutants through our work, as is the case for people involved with the plastics, dyestuffs, oil, asbestos, and atomic energy industries, but also those in the wood and solvents industries. These industrial pollutants lead to occupational cancers. The asbestos scandal is without doubt the most telling example. There was a reluctance to face up to the deleterious impact of asbestos on health for far too long. Industrial pollutants can also be found in water (seas, rivers, lakes, mineral waters, tap water, ground water) and in the food chain. The same is true of other products of manufacturing, including heavy metals (mercury, lead, etc.), polychlorinated biphenyls (PCBs), and parabens.

Throughout this book, we'll keep coming across such pollutants because with each day that goes by, they interfere more with what we eat, and to some extent, they also explain why what we ingest can be potentially carcinogenic.

Physical factors and heredity

Almost 5% of cancers are due to another environmental factor, either natural or unnatural in its cause. Radiation can come naturally from the sun (ultraviolet radiation, for example) or from the earth's natural radioactivity (radiation from the radon in the earth's crust). In the United States, the Environmental Protection Agency recommends that people get the radon radiation levels in their homes measured. Radioactivity produced by man (nuclear explosions, accidents in nuclear plants, etc.) is present in the atmosphere. Through rain and runoff it gets into the ground and into the plants produced on that ground (and into milk if the cow eats plants grown in radiation-tainted soil, as well as mushrooms, wild berries, etc.) and can last for many, many years. Here too, we can see that some carcinogenic effect reaches us through the food we eat.

Lastly, 5% of cancers are due to hereditary factors. Indeed, if all cancers are ultimately linked to an alteration in the genetic makeup of one of our cells (see *The Paths of Hope*),[14] in the vast majority of cases (95%) this alteration takes place during individuals' lifetimes and they will have received from their parents completely healthy and normal genes. Nevertheless, in rare cases (5%) some individuals inherit from their parents some genes that are already altered and already carry mutations likely to bring about the onset of a cancer. These cancers really are "hereditary." Even if these individuals lead a perfectly healthy life, they stand an enormous likelihood of developing a cancer, most often at a relatively young age.

So let's remind ourselves of the statement that although cancer is always a genetic disease, in the sense that it results from the effect of an abnormal gene, it is only very rarely a hereditary one (5%), in the sense that these abnormal genes are inherited from parents.

WE HAVE NOW ACCOUNTED FOR 80% of the causes of cancers: tobacco, hormones, infectious agents, pollution, physical factors, and heredity. We still have to clarify what causes the remaining 20% of cancers. And it's here where what we eat and drink comes into play.

THE CANCER ON OUR PLATES

Could feeding ourselves—eating and drinking—actually be responsible for 20% of human cancers? In fact, the percentage is probably far greater. We already mentioned some diet-related causes when we spoke of the pollution, radiation, and even infectious agents in our foods.

TABLE 1–4

**PROPORTION OF THE DIFFERENT CAUSES
IN THE RISK OF CANCER**

Cause of cancer	Estimated proportion
Tobacco	30%
Hormones	30%
Infectious agents	5%
Physical factors	5%
Genetic heredity factors	5%
Pollution	5%
Diet	20%

With little risk of getting it wrong, we may indeed claim that a good third of cancers are directly or indirectly linked to our diet.

So there's a whole wealth of possibilities for preventing cancer for us to consider. Unfortunately, what we are able to do is neither that obvious nor that simple to put in place, although we hope to make it more accessible in this book.

As it is, and contrary to what some people would like to have us believe, it's absolutely impossible to isolate the effect of any one specific food product. To arrogantly state that cutting out one particular food altogether—except for tobacco—or increasing our consumption of another food could prevent every single one of us from getting a specific cancer is total bunk!

If things were that simple, don't you think that from the time when cancer came and snatched our loved ones from us—for as long as humankind has existed—we would have gradually adopted life-saving habits? Or conversely, wouldn't we have abandoned any obviously carcinogenic behavior?

Just think about it for a moment. Without being a Nobel Prize winner for medicine, and given how hugely variable human beings are, how could you imagine that any one product could be good for all of us? Could the recommended quantities for foods be the same for a child of thirty pounds and for a man weighing almost two hundred pounds? For a woman who is at most risk of developing breast cancer and a man likely to develop prostate cancer?

Whatever our medical knowledge, we all know that we don't all digest foods in the same way. We don't all have the same metabolism, which is why even when following the very same diet, some people lose weight while others don't.

Whenever a study shows that a particular food is carcinogenic, have we taken the trouble to check whether the item is produced in exactly the same way as what we eat and whether it's prepared using the same cooking methods we use? Clearly not.

Some people would like us to take this type of oversimplified information at face value, which then means that it has no truth whatsoever for us. As we'll see, when we talk about red meat, for example—if we're being honest and want to protect ourselves properly—we can't dodge all the questions about where the meat came from, how the animals were fed and bred, how the meat was cooked, and how much of it we eat in one portion. Have our ages and therefore our nutritional requirements been taken into account, or our sex and consequently our metabolism (that is, what our bodies do with a product once we've ingested it)?

Finally, and most importantly, there are over twenty-five thousand bioactive compounds in the foods that the human race eats. Already over five hundred of these compounds have been identified as possible modulators of carcinogenesis.[15]

But we never eat a product on its own. Like all omnivores, our diet is always relatively diversified, not only what we eat throughout our lives, but also what we eat in the course of one meal. We practically never eat a meal made up of a single food.

We eat meat along with salt, bread, and vegetables. We have a starter beforehand, and we follow it sometimes with cheese or dessert. We use condiments, spices, and mustard. During the meal we drink something too. The examples could go on.

All these biocompounds in all these foods interact with one another and produce extraordinarily complex and varied combinations, which will similarly have extraordinarily complex and variable effects on our health. So let's stop seeing the carcinogenic risk from a meal as being purely the mathematical total of all the risks from each single item comprising the meal. That would be far too simple!

Likewise, these biocompounds are going to change chemically, depending on how the food is prepared and especially on how it's cooked. Are we sure that a grilled steak will have the same effect on our bodies as steak tartare? Or as stewed meat? Well, nothing could be less definite, and our intuition, always ahead of us, suggests as much.

You should be aware—and, as much as possible, this book will cover these points—that not only common sense but also scientific evidence confirms what our intuition very often suggests is true. If we wish to get close to the truth about the connection between what we eat and drink and cancer, we must first examine anything that might influence the complex relationships between these biocompounds and our bodies.

For our guidelines on what we need to do, we won't use studies carried out on a population that doesn't share the same characteristics and habits as our own, and therefore hasn't inherited the same exact enzymes as us. When a product has been tested but has nothing in common with an identically named product found elsewhere because its nutritional composition varies from one country to the next, we won't use the conclusions from such tests to work out recommendations for ourselves.

And whenever possible, we'll call upon our common sense, the common sense our mothers and grandmothers used, the common sense that over the centuries told them what they should give their children to eat to keep them healthy. These behavioral patterns enabled humankind, while respecting the limitations of a given biotope—that is, a certain environment—to grow, multiply, develop, adapt, and enjoy good health with far fewer cancers than in our current times.

Scientific data and general common sense

Where does all the information that we're going to discuss in this book come from? How do we know whether a particular food provides protection against cancer?

There are three major methods that allow us to get a handle on this sort of information: *epidemiological studies, experimental studies,* and *intervention studies on people.*[16]

However, before we tackle these methodologies, we'd like to let some of you make your own choice: to understand the "true anticancer diet," you don't have to read the next few pages. However, if you do want to understand the process by which we've reached a particular conclusion concerning the role of specific foods, then read these pages.

Let's start with *epidemiological studies.*

Epidemiological studies:
Case-control Studies and Cohort Studies

As far as the link between diet and cancer is concerned, there are two different types of studies, each with its own limitations. These are what we call "case-control" and "cohort" studies.

CASE-CONTROL STUDIES are by far the most common, since they are the easiest to carry out and the least expensive. They involve asking a group of cancer patients what they've eaten over a given period and then comparing the data with the answers obtained from a group of comparable but cancer-free individuals. If, for example, there's a marked difference with one food item, then it could bear some responsibility for the spread of the disease being studied.

You don't need to be a brilliant intellectual to immediately and intuitively grasp the immense limitations of this type of study. The subjects who are sick, the "test" subjects, just like the "control" subjects, can make mistakes when they try to recall what they've eaten at particular times in their life, especially with foods that are eaten only intermittently. They can fail to report eating another specific food at the same time (and this can change everything).

Moreover, the idea of individuals being comparable is, in itself, open to criticism. Obviously what is of interest to us is not the product in its natural state but what it turns into once it has been ingested, absorbed, metabolized, and distributed throughout the body and then excreted in the urine and stool. All these elements are likely to have an influence on whether a biocompound is carcinogenic. What really matters is how much of this biocompound, in its active form, actually reaches the cellular target and sets about turning a healthy cell into a cancerous one. And quite clearly this depends on the absorption, metabolism, distribution, and excretion that take place, which, in turn, depend on the individual's enzymes, which can vary hugely from one person to the next.

Take, for example, a food that may be carcinogenic if it remains in the mucous membrane of a particular organ for over two hours. If an individual absorbs this food but metabolizes it very quickly and then expels it through excretions, there is little likelihood of it causing cancer in this person.

Now imagine that genetically you are almost deficient in the enzymes that can metabolize and excrete this food. If you absorb the food, it'll linger for a long period in your body, with ample time to produce a harmful impact.

We can see how any variability of this sort can completely change the connection between a specific food and cancer. Yet, in these case-control studies, there's never any attempt to find out whether the two groups really are comparable in this way and if their metabolisms are identical.

Let's take another example to show how by simply overlooking one seemingly insignificant item of food, the outcome of a study can be totally altered. We know that vitamin D_3, which is found in dairy products, can, under experimental conditions, slow down growth in human cancer cells. (We'll come back to this later in the book.) We know that this is also true for genistein, which is found in soybeans and Sicilian pistachios.

However, when the two—vitamin D_3 and genistein—are combined in an experiment, the results are far better.[17] So, in theory at least, if the individuals in the study groups mention eating dairy products but forget to say that they also snacked on pistachios with their drink, any comparisons aiming to prove that milk protects us from cancer will be totally erroneous.

It can also happen that at the time a study is carried out, we are quite unaware of the existence of some specific risk factor for cancer totally unconnected with diet. If we don't yet know about it, we can't ensure that this factor is properly accounted for—that is, that it occurs with comparable frequency in both the test and the control groups.

Imagine having carried out a study on the role of a particular food and having established your conclusions about its link with the cancer in question, then discovering another factor that may potentially be responsible for this cancer. Because you knew nothing about the factor, however, you gave no consideration to it in your comparison. Your study is now invalid. You've no other choice but to start all over again, this time taking the new element into account.

This problem occurred recently in studies looking at the role wine plays in mouth cancers. At the time the studies on the link between drinking wine and oral cancers were carried out, nobody had any idea that most cancers of the mouth come from a virus, the human papillomavirus. As a result, since no researcher had checked any of the case-control studies to see whether the two groups being compared had equivalent oral-infection levels from the papillomavirus, these studies turned out to be unusable, and no results could be claimed.

Once again, just imagine for a moment that by pure chance more people in the heavy-wine-drinking group were carrying this virus but were unaware of it. This would mean that excessive wine consumption could no longer be held responsible for the greater incidence of oral cancers in this group, the greater incidence of this viral infection being instead to blame.

So we can see that for various reasons these studies, by far the most frequent, should be treated with great caution, and their conclusions should always be carefully scrutinized using clinical and common sense.

COHORT STUDIES are the second type of epidemiological study.

These studies are less common since they require a far greater investment of time and money. They involve following a large group of apparently healthy individuals and asking them to regularly fill in a record of what they eat. These individuals make up a "cohort" and have to be followed over a period of fifteen to twenty years to see whether any of them who develop a particular cancer had eating habits that varied from those individuals who remained in good health. Here again, it is fair to criticize how accurately the information is recorded and the possibility of some new carcinogenic factor appearing during the monitoring period or at the end of the study; significant biases are likely when the results are analyzed.

For example, imagine this time that when the cohort was set up twenty years ago, we had absolutely no inkling of the role turmeric could play in preventing stomach cancers, so that the subjects' records, which were routinely filled in, omitted any questions asking about it. Not only would we never have become aware of the role turmeric might play, but also if the individuals who ended up with stomach cancer had eaten less turmeric than the other participants, in all likelihood we'd have decided that they'd gotten this cancer because of a different factor, whereas the simple reason was that they hadn't eaten enough turmeric!

Experimental studies

These studies are far, far more worthwhile. They involve testing a specific product on cells in a culture or in animals. In addition, they enable us to work out the mechanisms by which a particular biocompound either has a carcinogenic effect or protects us from cancer, since these experiments can be conducted on cultivated cells in a laboratory.

We'll often refer to these studies in this book.

Experimental studies have their limitations too, which we'll try to take into consideration. When a food product is being tested, how this food is prepared or cooked is not generally taken into account. For example, if we take a vegetable that is usually eaten cooked and test the raw vegetable, will this raw vegetable produce the same effects as when we eat it in its cooked form?

Similarly, it's quite difficult to envisage testing all the possible food combinations that converge in all our various diets. Yet if this doesn't happen, we're likely to overlook the particular effect produced by one of these combinations.

The combination of products high in vitamin D and those in soybeans and pistachios was mentioned earlier. However, we could also mention the combination of turmeric with "piperine" (found in certain peppers), which boosts turmeric's effect.

Thus all these factors—the way foods are combined, prepared, and cooked—can help to modify or mask their carcinogenic or protective effects. So what can we do?

Intervention studies

These studies are the most complicated and the most expensive. They involve taking a large population of individuals, all quite healthy at the outset. This population is then divided into two completely comparable groups (we've already seen the limitations of doing this). All these individuals will then, every day, take pills that seem identical. For one of the two groups, the pills will contain a specific biocompound or a mix of biocompounds. The other group, without knowing it, will take placebo pills that contain, in other words, nothing at all.

All participants will be monitored over a designated number of years, after which they will be checked to see whether, as anticipated, the group taking the biocompound(s) does in fact show less incidence of a particular cancer than the other group. Such studies are few and far between, and we'll refer to them in our book whenever they can provide us with evidence that sheds light on our topic.

IS IT POSSIBLE TO EAT A DIET THAT PROTECTS US FROM CANCER?

For those of you who just read about the types of studies that are done, you'll understand the methodological principles that will enable us to critically analyze all the information presented. We'll know the right questions to ask, and we won't go blindly putting our faith in whatever some pseudo-specialist has to tell us. We'll realize each time that we not only have to try and find out where the information comes from, but also need to ask whether the study was done in the exact way needed to prove the hypothesis. We'll also know to check whether any consideration was given to how a product is produced and where it comes from (did you know, for example, that broccoli can contain from one to twenty-five times more glucoraphanin, the nutrient that actually protects us from cancer, depending on the variety?), how it is cooked and with what other foods, along with how we eat it, digest it, and excrete it. Lastly, but just as importantly, you need to ask whether this information applies to you depending on whether you're a woman or a man, whether you smoke or not, and whether you're a child or an adult.

As we've seen, the variability and the complexity of diets and their ramifications can be enormous. So let's be careful not to believe that simplification is possible and that generalizations or transpositions are acceptable.

Nothing could be less certain, which is why we should always bear in mind the notion of common sense. It has guided humankind unfailingly over thousands of years, and we'd like to believe that it's going to continue to do so for a long time to come. Let's allow common sense, along with the very best science, to guide us as we work our way through this book and the advice it contains.

Chapter 2

....

What Is Cancer?

....

WHERE DOES LIFE COME FROM?

Since we need to understand how the foods we eat can increase or decrease our risk of developing a cancer, I should explain to you how a cancer "works."

The very first thing you'll have to imagine is that any form of life or any living matter is composed of tiny building blocks that can fit together and multiply, what we call "cells." Human, animal, or plant, all living matter on our planet is made up of cells, with viruses being the only exception (we'll come back to this later). The simplest organisms, such as bacteria, are termed "unicellular" as they consist of a single cell. Most other living things—whether they belong to the animal or the vegetable kingdom, whether they live on land or in the sea—are the product of an extraordinarily precise and sophisticated collection of a multitude of cells. In fact, an adult human is made of approximately one million billion cells.

But where do these cells come from? Each living organism comes into being when a female cell (the ovum, the stamen, etc.) is fertilized by a male cell (the sperm, the pistil, etc.). These cells, one male and one female, once united, make up the first cell of a new individual. (I've simplified the science a touch because in reality both sex cells are only half-cells. Knowing this and how it is possible doesn't change or add anything to what I'm going to explain to you.)

At this stage, in your mother's womb, the human being you are about to become is contained in a single cell. This cell has a quite extraordinary feature that justifies it being called a "stem" cell. This characteristic makes the cell immediately capable of doing something amazing: the cell can make a copy of everything it contains—that is, it can multiply its intracellular material—and, once this is done, it can divide into two cells. Two cells are produced from one, and they are identical to each other, for now.

And so, little by little, day after day, these new cells will also, in turn, divide into two, following the same mechanism, giving birth each time to two cells from a single cell. These two cells will produce four. The four cells will produce eight, then sixteen, thirty-two, sixty-four, 128, 256, and so on. Living matter creating more living matter.

Before each division, each cell splits its material in two so that it can pass on the exact same inheritance, an inheritance that will be identical in every respect in the two cells it's about to produce. As this process unfolds, a phenomenon that we can call "quantitative," since it's all about increasing the quantity of living matter, of the cells, another astounding process gets under way. This is a more "qualitative" process.

These thousands, then, very quickly, millions of completely new cells, which in principle are all identical to each other, are going to start to "differentiate" themselves. In humans, some will turn into heart cells, others into kidney cells, and still others into brain cells or those of the liver, spleen, muscles, intestines, eyes, and so on. These differentiated cells will group together, according to their function, to make up organs.

By now, the original fertilized cell has developed into an embryo, and we can start to see the complex process taking shape that will make up a human body. Some cells will "organize themselves" into organs, which learn to function in harmony with one another. Gradually, a fetus and then a baby appears. This is the miracle of life!

Once this first cell is fertilized, it goes on to produce millions of billions of other cells. This multitude of cells will be part of a process, by the end of which each one of them will have taken on a single exclusive function (beating for cardiac cells, seeing for eye cells, digesting for stomach cells, and so forth). All the cells performing the same function will group together and then form organs. Each of these organs, following the example of each of the cells of which it is composed, will perform only one function. Thanks to all these organs that carry out their job fully and exclusively, an individual will be born, and will grow, develop, and live.

As long as we live, these processes will carry on even though a normal cell, no matter which organ it is in, is not eternal. Each cell lives for a few days or a few weeks and then dies.

Yet our organs remain functional. They regularly perform the task ascribed to them because just before each cell dies, as its life-span is coming to an end, it divides and gives birth to a completely new cell that replaces it. So, every day, around 70 million cells in our bodies die and 70 million are born. Except for the neurons in our brains, each time the aging cells realize that they're no longer performing their function well enough, because of senescence, they divide to give birth to new, youthful cells and then die to make way for them.

It is estimated, hold on now, that over a lifetime on average 10^{16} cell divisions take place—that is, 10,000,000,000,000,000 divisions! Aren't these figures astounding? However, if you're courageous enough to carry on reading this book, I'm going to give you some even more breathtaking figures shortly that will have you glued to your seat.

But let's get back to explaining cancer. So far, we've gone through the initial stage of understanding cancer by discussing where life comes from. There are three further stages. For me to explain—and for you to understand—how these quantitative phenomena of division and qualitative phenomena of differentiation are possible, we need to look inside the cell where the next stage takes place. To get the full picture, it will also be necessary for you to comprehend why a cell lives and carries out its function and why, when the time comes, it dies.

To grasp all this material, we need to think of the cell on a much smaller scale and get right inside it. We need to find out what is inside a cell and how a cell functions.

THE IMPORTANCE OF OUR GENES

In fact, what is inside a cell can be summarized quite simply without straying too far from the scientific reality, while at the same time simplifying the information sufficiently for it to make sense to those of you who haven't studied science. Roughly speaking, the interior of the cell contains a factory to produce proteins, a computer with the right programs to produce these proteins, and a power plant to provide energy.

Since we wish to understand how a cancer can come about, it's the "computer" that will be of prime interest to us. For this, we need to tell ourselves that a cell, which is there to perform a function, can perform that function only if it is told what to do. As amazing as a cell is, it can only do what its internal program commands it to do. In a similar way, if you don't have a word-processing program installed on your computer, it won't allow you to write anything at all. It's the same with our cells.

So then, what are these programs, or recipes, and where are they written inside the cell? Well, they are simply written into our chromosomes. Let's take our explanation a little further and get further inside the cell. Let's try to understand what our chromosomes are and how they work.

Chromosomes are our genetic material, our genes that are capable of defining us as a species and as an individual (think of the famous DNA or genetic fingerprinting in criminal investigations) and of giving our cells all the recipes they need to function properly.

Chromosomes, forty-six in humans, are made up of a substance called "DNA." This DNA is itself composed of a long chain that is coiled around itself when at rest and follows the linear assembly of four different molecules called organic bases ("bases" since they really are the basis of life). These four bases are designated by letters: A, T, C, and G. The four letters, the four bases, make up the genetic code, which was discovered almost sixty years ago by three amazing French researchers who won the Nobel Prize for that work: Dr. François Jacob, Dr. Jacques Monod, and Dr. André Lwoff.

These four letters (A, T, C, and G), joined to one another according to a very precise order, write into our DNA the thirty thousand genes that give us our characteristics and allow a million billion cells to function correctly, to divide, to differentiate themselves, to produce the proteins we need, and to live and die. In doing all this, they're fully responsible for whether we live or die. Bonded to one another, these bases—of which there are three billion in every one of our human cells—form a filament, which, brace yourselves, is two meters (six and a half feet) long and onto which our thirty thousand genes are written.

Let's go over this again, as it seems so utterly extraordinary. A human body is made up of a million billion cells, allocated (or differentiated) into two hundred different types, with each containing a two-meter-long filament onto which is written our thirty thousand genes using the three billion base molecules comprising the genetic code.

Try telling this to someone over dinner and see if they believe you! And yet it's true!

It gets even better: multiply what I've just told you by two. Each of our cells actually contains two filaments that are two meters long because one comes from the ovum and the other comes from the sperm. One gives us our mother's genes, the other our father's genes.

Even if all these numbers make you dizzy, they also help you to imagine just how tiny everything is that I'm talking about here, extraordinarily tiny, and therefore, as you might also expect, fragile.

All in all, we've grasped that these genes, which are the recipes from which all the components of life can be created, are written down with veritable letters, as if on a long parchment we call "DNA." Whenever a cell needs to make a protein that is necessary for it to perform its function, the cell unrolls this parchment and reads it until it reaches the gene required, and then it makes a sort of copy of this gene. Using a very sophisticated transport system, it sends this copy to the "protein factory." The required protein will then be produced, and the cell can perform its intended function.

Let's push on further with our desire to understand living matter.

We've said that genes are the programs that permit a cell to know how to do what it has to do. However, let's ask ourselves this question: What does a cell actually do?

In fact, cells have two actions. One is the proper action of all cells, whatever kind they are, which is to divide. The other is specific to each different type of cell, and that is to help the organ where the cell belongs to function.

Logically enough, there are two main types of genes in our DNA (in our chromosomes). Some genes regulate and control the process of division, and thus the life and death of the cell. Other genes carry the information needed to produce the functional proteins specific to each type of cell. You need to understand this point: each differentiated cell that belongs to and makes up a given organ assumes only one function. The cells in the heart beat so that the blood circulates, and those in the kidney produce urine to get rid of toxins. Imagine that one of them performed the task that the other was meant to do! The heart would produce urine, and the kidneys would start to beat!

Let's step up to a higher level of complexity. I promise you it's the final one. Alongside each of these genes, whether it's involved with cell division or cell function, there's also an "interrupter" or "promoter" gene. If it's touched, it activates the gene next to it, which will promote either division or the production of a protein.

Let's forget for now about the group of genes that code for functional proteins, and concentrate on the other genes, those for cell division and the promoters that control them.

Thus, we have now arrived at the point I wanted us to reach: a cancer is almost always the result of damage to one of these genes.

How is this possible?

CANCER IS A GENETIC DISEASE

If a gene responsible for cell division and cell multiplication is damaged, or if there is damage to the promoter genes that under normal circumstances switch it on or off, then we have a disaster. The multiplication of the cell is no longer under control; it is no longer regulated. It no longer functions according to need, but instead becomes anarchic. The cell divides, and then it divides again and again. It goes out of control, like a car without brakes racing ahead at top speed. One cell produces two, then four, then eight, sixteen, thirty-two, sixty-four, and so on. These cells multiply endlessly, and, provided they can find enough food to ensure their survival, nothing is able to stop their proliferation. They multiply like crazy, and soon this becomes deadly for their host. They quickly form a lump, a tumor. This tumor will swell and invade the adjoining tissues, disrupting their function. The invaded organs suffer and then become incapable of performing their functions. But these malignant cells couldn't care less about all that. They continue to divide, producing ever more cells until this infernal process is no longer compatible with the individual's life.

To fully grasp just how devastating this phenomenon is, you need to realize that a tumor measuring one centimeter (just over one-third of an inch) in diameter already contains one billion cancerous cells all clustered together, all developed from this initial cell where, one day, the genes controlling its ability to divide were impaired.

It's as simple as that, and as terrible!

One can, at the end of this second stage that we've just looked at, say that a cancer is almost always caused by the uncontrolled multiplication of a cell in which the genes that normally regulate its capacity to divide have become damaged and altered.

Come on! Just two more stages to go, and then we'll talk about diet.

Damaged genes

With this next stage, we'll understand how it is that these particular genes can become damaged. I'll tell you straightaway, it's this final stage that will allow us to envision the molecular processes that explain the effect foods have on the state of these famous genes.

At the point we're at now, we're trying to answer the question of how these genes can get damaged. In getting to this stage of the book, you'll have well understood that our genes really are texts written with "real" letters, even if these four letters are chemical molecules. These provide a true and tangible organic material that takes the shape of two coiled filaments parallel to one another, the DNA that we learned to call "chromosomes" at school.

Quite simply, we can think back to how there is the potential risk of a mistake occurring right before every cell divides into two daughter cells and the DNA has to be duplicated. If you remember, just before a cell divides into two, it must duplicate itself, splitting in half its intracellular material and, most importantly, its genetic material. This process is fundamental since it guarantees that from one cell to the next, the proper characteristics of each species are preserved and, within the species, those of each individual.

To say it one more time, as we've already seen, a cell is what its genes tell it to be. It does what its genes tell it to do. In other words, it's a human cell because it contains, just like each cell of its kind, the thirty thousand genes of the human species.

Thus, it is imperative that each living cell carry out the synthesis —the production—of an absolutely (and when I say absolutely, I really do mean absolutely) identical copy of its DNA, of its genes, so that before it divides, the material it will give to both cells—that is, to the two cells it's going to produce—is of the exact same genetic inheritance, the exact same chromosomes.

Let's look at an example so that we get a better grasp of why this is really crucial. You all know that the color of our eyes or skin is genetically determined—that is, programmed and controlled by our genes. Now imagine that you've got blue eyes and fair skin, but that, cell division after cell division, your cells don't keep your genetic makeup identical, which means, in particular, that the genes that make your eyes blue and your skin fair do not remain stable. What will happen? Little by little, your eyes will change color and turn brown, for example; likewise, your skin will get darker. In this case, after a certain amount of time, you will no longer really be yourself, at least if you compare yourself to the picture and personal details recorded on your passport or photo ID.

This example is very simplistic, but I hope it helps you understand how the quality of the copy of our genes, which is made before each cell division, is crucial. If the copy isn't complete, profound changes can occur in our bodies.

Fortunately for us, this process to produce an identical copy is usually very efficient, bordering on perfection. So don't worry, tomorrow you'll look just the same as you do today. Still . . . this feat has to be repeated seventy million times a day, that's over eight hundred times a second, without there ever being the slightest mistake for your whole life, whereas, as we've already seen, there are 10,000,000,000,000,000 (10^{16}) opportunities in a lifetime for a mistake to creep in.

Moreover, this mistake doesn't even need to be quantitatively very significant. It could simply be a case of one of these four letters from the genetic alphabet being written in place of another letter. Of all the three billion letters that one of our DNA filaments contains, it could be just one letter, so tiny and so fragile—just a T instead of a C or an A—and perhaps the whole meaning of the "word" in the "text" will actually change. An interrupter gets switched on that is meant to be switched off. A gene that blocks division in a normal situation now doesn't block it. Or, conversely, a gene that is meant to activate division only a little bit gets carried away and activates it like crazy.

One simple, tiny letter where another is meant to be. An unfortunate substitution. An error with one molecule measuring less than a billionth of a millimeter, and yet this can result in the emergence of mortal danger: a cell that starts to divide, reproduce, and multiply itself endlessly, without control, without reason, without the body having a need for it. This one cell produces monstrous descendants, famished cells, which take over the area they are in need of, attacking other cells and destroying other organs. Death spreads and advances, blinded by a gene for which, quite simply, one letter was badly written.

I'll just mention in passing that, luckily for us, when we make spelling mistakes, the repercussions aren't quite so catastrophic.

Cancer is not inevitable

But let's return to this cell, which, while preparing a copy of its text so it can divide, has just made a mistake, which we term a "mutation."

As we've come to realize, given the number of cell divisions, it's impossible for this catastrophic scenario not to occur thousands of times in each and every one of us throughout our lives.

What happens then? Does a cancer appear every time? Happily, no. Otherwise, we'd all be long dead from this disease.

Luckily, nature foresaw the possibility of DNA mutating. To avoid the serious consequences that would arise each time this happens, nature devised a whole system to verify the inscription of our genes—a careful reading, if you prefer, of the three billion bases of our DNA— and, in case it detected an error, a mutation, a whole second system to correct and repair it.

What's more, equally likely as these mutations are those that can occur at times other than during the synthesis phase prior to cell division. In fact, DNA is also permanently exposed to the risk of being damaged by the effect of certain physical or chemical phenomena. If you wanted to keep count, it's estimated that over ten thousand DNA mutations take place daily in each of our cells.

For example, we now know that when they're functioning, the protein factory and power plant in our cells produce chemical molecules capable of reacting with the DNA bases and causing considerable damage to the DNA filament. For those of you who'd like to know more, there are the examples of hydrogen peroxide, hydroxyl radicals, or the very reactive compounds of oxygen that are called "free radicals." These radicals, normally very corrosive to DNA, are the products of cellular metabolism—that is, they are part of the lifecycle of the cell. These radicals are permanently detoxified within the interior of the cell before they can even reach the DNA. However, just like everything else in this world, this detoxification system doesn't always work perfectly. A hyperactive free radical can reach the DNA, react chemically with a base (A, T, C, or G), and destroy it. Is it really that important if one letter among three billion goes missing? If this happened with an enormous book, a novel with three billion letters, you probably wouldn't even notice. But when dealing with something as delicate and subtle as life—with the genes that determine our life and our death—it can be catastrophic.

These mutations can also be caused by factors outside the cell, such as radiation that reaches us and sometimes penetrates inside us (ultraviolet rays, radiation from radioactivity, etc.) or foods that interfere with the DNA's synthesis processes (we'll look at this later). Here again, the probability that this will never happen—that the control systems will let nothing past them, that the detoxification system will work correctly at every single moment, that the repair systems, too, will never ever make a single mistake while repairing all these mutations—is nil.

These errors, these malfunctions, and these accidents do occur. And each time they generate the possibility of a malignant, cancerous cell emerging. One cell among a million billion other cells that are normal. But the cells that this abnormal cell produces will grow larger day by day and end up casting aside life's harmony as it ushers in death. Alongside the processes that control cell division, we can see how crucial these DNA repair systems are when it comes to cancer risks.

We won't look at how these DNA repair mechanisms work. To keep it simple, just remember that there are several types and that they correspond to the different types of possible damage to our genetic material. The repair systems the cells resort to will not necessarily be the same. The system employed will depend on whether there's an extra letter (or group of letters), a missing letter, or a letter that has gotten swapped with another one. However, ultimately all these systems share a common, fundamental, and unique goal: to preserve our DNA's stability and integrity for the life of a cell and for each of our cells as long as we live.

So, well done! You've just followed and, I hope, understood what I have to admit is a fairly high-level lesson on molecular biology. If you've managed to grasp everything I've just explained, you know more or less as much as a young medical student.

Now, perhaps, you ought to put the book down for a few minutes so you can relax and think about something else before we go on to tackle the final phase in this chapter: the connection between the processes I've just described and our food and drink.

NUTRIGENOMICS: THE CONNECTION BETWEEN OUR DIET AND CANCER

We've come to understand that when the genetic makeup of one of our cells suffers a loss of integrity, cancer is almost always the result. Unrepaired or badly repaired abnormalities appear, carried by one or several genes, which in normal circumstances would control and regulate the processes of cell division that are indispensable to all forms of life.

These genes, fundamental both to life and paradoxically to cancer, again also fall into two main types. Here, I'll just run through them very briefly, as their only interest for us is as possible targets for the pro-carcinogenic or anticarcinogenic workings of our foods. There are two types: the genes that stimulate cell division and those that inhibit it. The first type, the accelerator, is called an "oncogene" because if it is abnormally activated, it brings about a malignant tumor. The second type, the brake, is called a "tumor-suppressor gene" or an "anti-oncogene," since it does the opposite: when it is activated, it blocks cell multiplication and therefore stops cancer from developing.

Among these cancer genes, some are worth getting to know a little better. Let's start with oncogenes. To stimulate or promote cellular multiplication, most of the oncogenes need to know the code—that is, they need to have the recipe for the protein "duos" called "growth factors," which, as their name suggests, act just like fertilizers. These duos are made up of both a receiver protein (the receptor), which is fixed to the cell's surface—on its outer membrane, or skin if you like—and a messenger protein (the growth factor), which is consigned to the exterior of the producer cell and will look for its specific receptor. If the producer cell finds its receptor, it becomes precisely embedded in it. This full, complete contact between the receptor and its matching messenger sets off a signal inside the cell to which the receptor is fixed. A little like when someone rings the doorbell, this signal spreads inside the cell through a series of cascading reactions, which we well understand now. It finishes upon reaching the interrupters of the division genes (the ones we saw earlier), which then get switched on, causing cell multiplication.

One of the tumor-suppressor genes (anti-oncogenes), the p53 or the "guardian of the genome," is more important than the others, so we need to know about it. As previously mentioned, it is crucial for a cell's genome to remain complete. We've also seen that there's a multiple-reading system for the genome—for the two DNA filaments—and that a repair process is implemented if an abnormality is detected.

The DNA is permanently read and reread, like a music CD you play continually on your player. Imagine then that among the thirty thousand genes, there's one gene, the p53, whose role is to listen to this music. As long as it hears that the DNA is untouched (that there's no false note in the music), it does nothing. On the other hand, if at any time, as usually happens when the cell is growing old and its repair systems are not particularly efficient, the p53 hears that what should have been harmonious music has turned into a veritable cacophony and that problems with the genome are no longer being properly repaired, it quickly directs the cell to commit suicide, called "apoptosis." Rather than running the risk of allowing this cell to become a danger to the other cells, the p53 gene prefers that the cell commit suicide, even though that will also kill the p53 gene in the cell.

Once again, we see that if a cell produces too many receptors capable of stimulating its growth, or some overly sensitive receptors, or even stimulating messengers ("growth factors" in medical language) in too great a quantity, then a cancer will likely be produced. For example, if the p53 or other anti-oncogenes no longer function because of a mutation, and changes to the genome could be produced, there would be a fatal change at one moment or another, one conducive to the multiplication of malignant cells.

At this time, what do we know about the general principles influencing the connections between genes, cancer, and nutrition?

The science that studies these connections is called "nutrigenomics." Although admittedly still a fledgling science, a certain number of studies are beginning to be published, and they already point to some interesting leads, even if they aren't yet absolute certainties.

In order to understand why this science is so important and why I thought it was time for me to write this book, we can appeal one more time, quite simply, to common sense.

WE NOW KNOW THAT EACH CELL in our body must make a full set of forty-six chromosomes more than eight hundred times every second. From this point of view, to produce an object, whether it be on the infinitesimally small scale of a cell or on a much larger scale, two things are necessary: materials and energy.

The same goes for any cell that wants to divide. First, though, it has to make chromosomes. For this, it also needs energy and materials. It only has a single way to produce this energy: it makes it by burning sugar.

Unlike us, the cell can't choose whether to burn wood, coal, or kerosene or whether to turn to nuclear or hydraulic power. No, a cell can only produce energy from burning one thing: sugar. Either the cell burns sugar that has just been eaten or it uses sugar that has been stored by the body in different forms to cope with shortages. To burn this sugar, it also needs oxygen. Fresh blood continuously sends a supply of oxygen to the cell. The hemoglobin found in red blood cells transports the oxygen and also gives blood its color.

Sugar and oxygen—these are the basic elements required for energy to be produced in our cells. I mean normal cells. And in all our cells.

The materials for cell division are composed of two other types of basic nutrients: proteins and fats. The fats—lipids—can also be transformed into sugar if the need arises, and can then be used for the combustion just mentioned. Proteins are really the basic elements or materials used to build all living matter.

Imagine you had to build a house. You need bricks (proteins), energy (sugars), and, between the two, lipids, which get used either to provide energy or to alter the proteins to give them specific properties that are vital for their function.

In addition to these three basic components, to ensure that the different parts of the house are solid, efficient, and beautiful, you need components such as trace elements, metals, and lots of very simple molecules to serve as the cement, glue, and electric wires. These materials will cause, catalyze, and control certain reactions that are essential to the cell functioning correctly.

Now, I have a simple question for you: Where do all these products come from—these proteins, lipids, carbohydrates, vitamins, and other trace elements? The simple answer is that they come from what we eat. And the oxygen comes from the air we breathe.

If we don't eat good-quality food, or if we eat an unbalanced diet or food that doesn't fit our needs (which vary from one person to the next; we'll return to this), what we eat and drink will provide us with bad building materials, and our cell synthesis processes may get disrupted. We build our cells with what we eat, of course.

And that isn't all. In addition to what our common sense would have told us anyway, we now know that the biocompounds in our food can also work directly on the DNA repair processes; on the cell differentiation mechanisms; on our genes' state of reactivity, or, alternatively, on sending our genes to sleep; and even on the production of internal carcinogens, or, conversely, on their detoxification. And, finally, they act directly on our DNA's capacity to prepare itself to be duplicated in the synthesis phase that precedes any division.

And that's nutrigenomics.

All that!

In other words, nutrigenomics is a science about food materials. It is also about how foods can stimulate, block, and prepare the particular chemical reactions that may play an absolutely crucial role in carcinogenesis.

THE EFFECTS OF FOOD BIOCOMPOUNDS

Before looking at the effect of different foods, I thought it would be interesting to give you a few ideas about the effects of some food biocompounds on the various key systems that regulate cell proliferation. I intend to talk about the systems for DNA repair, activation of our genes, promotion of differentiation, and, finally, production of carcinogenic toxins and their detoxification, respectively.

We know, for example, that as a rule, malnutrition lessens our capacity to repair DNA and, conversely, that fruits like kiwis or trace elements such as selenium boost it. It has even been shown quite recently that juices with a high lycopene content markedly improve the activity of these systems.

We also know that there are different degrees of ability to activate a gene. If it can't be activated at all, we then say the gene has been made silent. In this case, nothing will be able to activate it. A few carbon and hydrogen atoms stuck to the molecules surrounding the gene are all it takes to silence it.

In nature this process is often used to prevent dangerous genes, and oncogenes can be dangerous, from getting activated too often. This process is dependent on two types of antagonist enzymes. The enzymes that silence genes are histone acetyltransferases (HATs). The enzymes that do the opposite are histone deacetylases (HDACs).

So we now know that certain substances will inhibit HDACs, thereby lowering the risk of cancer. This is true for the butyrate produced when certain polysaccharides ferment in the intestines, and for the diallyl disulfide found in garlic and the sulforaphane in cabbage.[1]

As for the differentiation mechanisms that tend to lower the cells' capacity to multiply, nowadays we know that retinoic acid by-products found, for example, in carrots and certain polyunsaturated fatty acids particularly common in fish oils can stimulate it and act as fantastic anticancer agents.[2]

Lastly—and this is one of the most exciting areas of nutrigenomics —as we round off this general-background chapter, we need to talk about the mechanisms that produce carcinogenic toxins and detoxification for these products.

Not only in what we eat and in what we drink, but also inside our bodies, owing to the natural functioning of our organs, there are some substances that can become carcinogenic if they are affected by metabolic bioactivation: to some extent, our bodies make some quite carcinogenic substances. The enzymes that can produce them are called "phase I" enzymes, and they are present in varying degrees from one individual to another. These enzymes may also be more or less active and therefore produce more or fewer carcinogens.

Everything about them, whether we have them or not and whether they are active or not, is genetically determined: this means that whether we have many of these enzymes or not and whether they're underactive or hyperactive is inherited from our parents. These enzymes, of which cytochrome p450, peroxidases, and transferases are the most well known, explain why some smokers develop lung cancer while others do not.

It's these enzymes that produce highly carcinogenic substances from the tobacco smoke.[3] So if you happen to have a lot of these enzymes, even if you smoke only a little, you'll produce large quantities of carcinogenic substances and have a high risk of getting lung cancer. Conversely, if you don't have these enzymes or have very few, you may well be able to smoke without too great a risk.

This reasoning holds true for all situations in which our bodies come into contact with polycyclic hydrocarbons, for example, from overcooked meat or meat cooked over a flame, or with other substances that may be found in foods, such as aflatoxins, which nowadays, fortunately, are very rarely found in nuts. It has been proved that grapefruit juice, garlic, and red wine can inhibit these "phase I" enzymes, thereby lessening our risk of getting cancer.[4]

On the other hand, the enzymes that detoxify carcinogenic products and enable us to expel them before they can do us harm are called "phase II" enzymes. Glutathione S-transferase is one of the most common. Once these enzymes act, they really do detoxify most potentially carcinogenic compounds.

Phase II enzymes are stimulated by the isothiocyanates found in foods like Brussels sprouts and red cabbage (but not in white cabbage or broccoli).[5]

FROM READING THE ABOVE, we've realized through common sense or scientific experimentation why there's bound to be a connection between what we eat and our risk of getting a cancer. We've seen how and why this connection exists.

We've even started to get a foretaste of what we need to do and what it is best to avoid doing in regard to cancer. We've looked at all this in quite some depth, which at this stage might have frightened some of you. I'd like to reassure you, we went through all this background so that I could show you that everything I'm going to tell you is serious. I've thought much about what I want to say, accumulating knowledge and testing out common sense over a long time.

Everything that now follows will be easy to read; there won't be any more scholarly words. We'll simply talk about foods and how we can feed ourselves better so as to lower our risk of one day developing a cancer. We'll start by examining the main food groups and then finish off by giving you our "anticancer advice."

Please don't listen to anyone who tells you that a single diet can be right for everyone, that a diet can be equally suitable for young women whose bodies are full of female hormones (potentially highly carcinogenic for their breasts) as for menopausal women whose bodies hardly secrete hormones any more. Or that the same diet can be just as appropriate for heavy smokers, who each day need to repair the millions of injuries inflicted on their DNA by the carcinogens in their cigarettes, as it is for others who don't smoke at all.

Since that can't be true, the excellent nutritionist Nathalie Hutter-Lardeau and I have endeavored to give you genuine "à la carte" anticancer advice. So, together, and without further ado, let's take a closer look at the foods in our diet.

Chapter 3

········

Is Fish a Health Food or a Health Risk?

···

A s we now take a look at all the different foods, let's start off with fish.

We couldn't help but start here as by definition fish is nowadays symbolic of "good for your health" food. Often compared to meat, which we'll examine later, the nutritional value of fish is supposed to be top quality: it's full of proteins, omega-3, the polyunsaturated fats that we all know help tackle depression,[1] and yet it contains relatively few calories.

TABLE 3-1

CLASSIFICATION OF FISH ACCORDING TO FAT CONTENT[2]

	Fat content	Fish
Oily fish	> 5%	Raw or smoked salmon, mackerel, herrings, sardines, anchovies, halibut, swordfish
Semi-oily fish	1–5%	Bass, turbot, tuna, mullet
Lean fish	< 1%	Cod, sole, smoked haddock, sea bream, hake, skate

DOES FISH HELP PROTECT
AGAINST CANCER?

Our image of fish is of a natural creature that feeds freely on the food it finds in the seas, without any intervention from humans, swimming in immense oceans that are far less polluted than our land, unaffected by any notion of yield, genetic modification, or degradation through humankind's folly.

We are so taken with this idea that in the United States the average individual annual consumption has gone from 11.0 pounds in 1950–59 to 15.2 pounds in 2000, an increase of almost 50% in fifty years.

In the year 2000, 2.6 billion humans (43% of the world's population) fed themselves primarily on fish, and furthermore, to a greater or lesser extent, they lived from catching or farming it.[3]

It is indeed true that when we look at what's in fish, it may appear to be a top-quality, natural food. But does this necessarily mean that eating it regularly will prevent us from getting cancer?

Not really, or, in any case, not much. When all of the studies that have attempted to show that eating significant amounts of fish is beneficial with regard to certain cancers are analyzed, the results suggest that at most it might lower the risk of only colon cancer, and that by only 3% or 4%.[4]

In other words, as far as having a beneficial effect goes, it's very negligible indeed.

However, to my mind, nowadays we really should be asking this question the other way around: Is there any risk in us eating more fish as we are tending to do?

Here is where this question gets answered in part. In 2005, the Environmental Protection Agency (EPA), the organization responsible for protecting American's health and the environment, published data about the contamination in fish from coastal waters. Then in 2009, the agency published further data on the contamination of fish in American lakes and reservoirs. The results show that persistent organic pollutants (POPs) and other contaminants are very widespread. Mercury and polychlorinated biphenyls (PCBs) were detected, in lesser or greater amounts, in all the samples of fish, which were taken from five hundred American lakes and reservoirs. As for the fish taken from coastal waters (including the Great Lakes), more than one in five was highly contaminated, with PCBs being the main contaminant, followed by mercury. Moreover, it's important to note that in 2010, 98% of the fish advisories issued by the local authorities regarding fish consumption involved five bioaccumulative chemical compounds: mercury, PCBs, chlordane, dioxins, and DDT. And as for arsenic, in general, it's present in more than 50% of seafood products across the world. (See Tables 3-3(a) to 3-3(d).)[5]

In another study carried out by the World Health Organization (WHO), 99% of methylmercury,[6] the most toxic mercury compound that the population takes in on a daily basis, comes primarily from eating fish.[7]

Certain fish, and later we'll see which ones and why, are so contaminated by these metals that at times we could actually think of them as mineral deposits! This wouldn't necessarily be of any grave concern if these products hadn't been classified as "proven to be carcinogenic" to humans by the WHO's International Agency for Research on Cancer (IARC).[8] (See Table 3-2.) In fact, nowadays, quite often if you're not careful, when you think you're eating fish, in actual fact you're taking in serious amounts of heavy metals.

Fortunately, however, contamination varies from one species of fish to another, and it also varies according to where the fish comes from.[9] To avoid getting contaminated or contaminating your children, you have to chose carefully and develop the right habits.

The EPA has made available to the public a compendium of information on locally issued fish advisories and safe eating guidelines. This information is provided to the EPA by states, U.S. territories, Indian tribes, and local governments, which issue advisories and guidelines to inform people about the recommended level of consumption for fish caught in local waters.

Pollutants in the sea

But, first, let's take a look at some carcinogenic contaminants. Most have been mentioned already: mercury, lead, dioxin, PCBs, and arsenic.

Unfortunately, this list is far from being exhaustive. For many years we've been polluting our oceans, our fish have become polluted from them, and in turn we've been polluting ourselves by eating this seafood. And there's a huge number of these pollutants.

A major problem with these pollutants, which we ingest and which accumulate inside our bodies, is that they take a very long time to disappear. For example, the biological half-life of cadmium is thirty

TABLE 3-2

AGENTS CLASSIFIED BY THE INTERNATIONAL AGENCY FOR RESEARCH ON CANCER (IARC) (NON-EXHAUSTIVE LIST)[10]

IARC Classification	Agent listed
Carcinogenic to humans (group 1)	Arsenic, asbestos, cadmium, *H. pylori*, aflatoxins, salted fish, tobacco, benzene, benzo[a]pyrene, chromium [VI], estrogen-progestogen menopausal therapy, nonsteroidal estrogens, ethanol, hepatitis B virus, hepatitis C virus, human papillomavirus, radon, solar radiation, betel, coal tar, household combustion of coal
Probably carcinogenic to humans (group 2A)	Acrylamide, inorganic lead, PCBs, frying emissions from high temperatures, hot yerba mate, androgens, 5-methoxypsoralen, nitrates and nitrites, ultraviolet (UV) radiation encompassing UVA, UVB, and UVC, non-arsenical insecticides
Possibly carcinogenic to humans (group 2B)	Coffee, chlorophenoxy herbicides, lead, nickel, pickles
Not classifiable as to its carcinogenicity to humans (group 3)	Acrolein, Evans blue, caffeine, native carrageenin, cholesterol, chlorinated drinking water, glass-wool insulation, mercury and its mineral compounds, paracetamol, quercetin, saccharin, sulfites, tea
Probably not carcinogenic to humans	Caprolactam

TABLE 3-3(A)

MERCURY LEVELS IN FISH AND SHELLFISH

Species	Mercury Level (ppm)		Number of samples
	Mean	Maximum	
Bigeye tuna	0.689	1.816	21
Bluefish	0.368	1.452	94
Grouper	0.448	1.205	53
Halibut	0.241	1.205	53
Lobster	0.166	0.451	71
Mackerel	0.730	1.670	213
Marlin	0.485	0.920	16
Oyster	0.012	0.250	61
Salmon	0.022	0.190	94
Scallop	0.003	0.083	90
Shark	0.979	4.540	356
Shrimp	0.009	0.050	40
Snapper	0.166	1.366	67
Squid	0.023	0.070	42
Swordfish	0.995	3.220	636
Tilefish (Gulf of Mexico)	1.450	3.730	60

TABLE 3-3(B)

CADMIUM LEVELS IN FISH AND SHELLFISH

Species	Cadmium level (µg/100 g), up to
Bluefish	0.08 FW
Blue marlin	83 FW
Clam	39.8 DW
Cod	0.09 DW
Lobster	33.8 DW
Mussel	18.2 DW

Species	Cadmium level (µg/100 g), up to
Oyster	9.0 DW
Red abalone	1163 DW
Scallop	546.6 DW
Shrimp	6.4 DW
Squid	782 DW
Striped bass	0.3 FW
Yellowtail flounder	0.4 DW

Note: DW, dry weight; FW, Fresh weight.

TABLE 3-3(C)

LEAD LEVELS IN FISH AND SHELLFISH

Species	Lead level (µg/100 g), up to
Common carp	12 DW
Crawfish	500 DW
Sea urchin	58 DW
Shrimp	24 DW
Fish, whole, nationwide	1.9 FW
U.S. coastal marine fishes	3 FW

Note: DW, dry weight; FW, fresh weight.

TABLE 3-3(D)

CONTAMINANTS IN COASTAL FISH TISSUES IN 48 LAKES AND RESERVOIRS OF THE CONTIGUOUS UNITED STATES, COMPARED WITH HEALTH-BASED GUIDELINES, 1997–2000

Contaminant	Guideline range (Concentration, in ppm)	Percentage of estuarine site exceeding guideline range
Arsenic (inorganic)	3.5–7.0	0
Mercury (muscle tissue)	0.12–0.23	18
Total PCBs	0.023–0.047	19
DDT	0.059–0.120	8

years, and for dioxin it ranges from seven to eleven years,[11] quite enough time to wreak its dreadful, carcinogenic effect.[12]

PCBs deserve a special mention. They appeared in the industrial world around 1930. Deemed extremely harmful, they stopped being produced in 1987. Since they are nonflammable, PCBs were widely used to manufacture condensers and transformers, but they were also used for paints, insulating material, soldered joints, and more. There are over two hundred PCBs; some are more toxic than others.[13] These products don't evaporate, and they don't dissolve in water because, most of the time, they are insoluble. However, they are liposoluble (that is, soluble in fats), which explains why they are found accumulated in fish tissue and fish fat.

The more a species is a carnivorous predator, the higher up it is in the food chain and the more likely it is to be contaminated.[14] Moreover, this phenomenon holds true for most POPs, which are hardly biodegradable at all.

So you can now understand why of all the fish species, salmon, red

TABLE 3-4

PCB CONTENT PER PRODUCT GROUPS[15]

Products	PCB content (mg/100 g of raw product)
Cephalopods (octopuses, squid)	450
Shellfish	730
Crustaceans (lobsters, etc.)	180
Average contamination for all seafood	420
Freshwater fish (except eels)	3,020
Freshwater oily fish (> 2%)	5,570
Freshwater lean fish (< 2%)	1,960
Eels	24,100
Farmed fish	1,120
Saltwater oily fish (> 2%)	2,880
Saltwater lean fish (< 2%)	760
Average contamination for all fish	1,890

tuna, and swordfish, which are high up on the food chain and are fatty fishes, are most dangerous for our health.

If you've seen the movie *Erin Brockovich*, you might remember that it is based on what happened in the town of Anniston, Alabama, where between 1929 and 1971, thirty-two thousand tons of PCBs were disposed of in an open public dumpsite. We have two further examples from recent history of massive human contamination from PCBs. In 1968 in Japan and then in 1979 in Taiwan, accidental leakage of PCBs occurred in rice-oil factories. Thousands of people were contaminated via their food, and on both occasions this led to a multitude of cancers.[16]

Meal after meal, our bodies are being poisoned

We can see that regardless of where PCBs, heavy metals, and POPs come from, they're toxic for our health and significantly increase our risk of cancer.[17] We've also seen that our intake of heavy metals and POPs is primarily due to our ingesting seafood and products made from it.

Furthermore, Dr. J. A. Davis, from the San Francisco Estuary Institute, wrote in 2007, "However, 25 years after the ban, PCB concentrations in some Bay sport fish today are still more than 10 times higher than the Threshold of Concern."[18] What's true for PCB concentrations in the fish in San Francisco Bay is generally true for a certain number of fish and shellfish in the United States as a whole. So as Dr. E. Oken and the Harvard Medical School team wrote in 2012, "Fish provides a rich source of protein and other nutriments, but because of contaminations by methylmercury and other toxicants, higher fish intake often leads to greater toxicant exposure."[19]

What we need to really grasp is that apart from intentional dumping or accidents, of which a few notable examples have been mentioned, we're dealing here with long and repeated exposure, day after day, in small doses each time we absorb carcinogenic compounds by eating fish. Meal after meal, these substances, which are hardly biodegradable, accumulate inside our bodies, in our liver, in our brains, in our fatty tissues, and in our blood. The fear is that repeated ingestion of these substances upsets our metabolic processes and over the long term encourages the development of cancers.

A Spanish study conducted in 2004, by a team from the Barcelona university hospital, proved that PCBs play a leading role in creating cancerous tumors in the colon.[20] A Swedish study showed that cancers of the pancreas, dreadful enough as they start out become even more serious with any exposure to Pyralenes (a commercial name for PCBs).[21]

But who reads these studies? Who talks about them? Another study carried out by the French Association of Environmental Health (ASEF) aroused my interest. Fifty-two volunteers living on the banks of the Rhône, close to high-polluting, large industrial facilities, were asked to give blood samples so that the PCB content could be measured. Those who regularly ate local fish had very high PCB levels at times (up to 93 pg/g, which is colossal).[22]

SHOULD ALL FISH BE BANNED?

Certainly not. The studies show that the risk of contamination depends on the breed of fish and where it is caught. In France, there's a survey (CALIPSO) that lets consumers know the degree of contamination for each type of fish according to the port where it is caught.[23] We haven't found such an exhaustive survey covering fish in the United States, except for the EPA report already mentioned.

Indeed, when some people state that we need to ingest omega-3 to avoid getting cancer, which has not actually been proved, we are being faced with an apparently difficult choice: Do we eat more fish high in omega-3 while at the same time swallowing more highly carcinogenic pollutants and metals, or do we avoid these serious cancer-producing substances but then do without omega-3?

Fortunately, with a clearer understanding of the facts, we can perhaps find a solution. As we've said, the fish with the highest levels of mercury are predator fish, such as swordfish, marlin, red tuna, and eels.[24] Even if they do contain beneficial nutrients, you should avoid them. However, there are other types of fish, also high in omega-3, that generally contain far less mercury, such as mackerel, anchovies, and sardines.

Be careful and check where your fish and your shellfish come from, so you can work out how to select the ones that are the least contaminated. Protect your health by being far more selective when buying seafood than you have been in the past. Furthermore, take heed of the French Food Safety Agency, which knows what it is talking about when, in its latest official guidelines, it recommends that as far as predator fish are concerned, pregnant women should not exceed one 5-oz. (150-g) portion per week and children under 2½ years no more than 2 oz. (60 g) per week.[25] Likewise, in the United States, American authorities know what is right too. Starting in 2004, the EPA and Food and Drug Administration (FDA) issued joint recommendations about limiting the amount of fish eaten by specific sectors of the population—pregnant and breastfeeding women and young children—with the aim of reducing their exposure to the harmful effects of mercury. They advocate avoiding the fish most contaminated with mercury (for example, swordfish, shark) and limiting consumption of less contaminated species to twice a week (that is, 12 oz. per week in total). They also suggest that you ask local authorities of the probable mercury contamination before eating any fish caught nearby and if no information is available, then eat no more than 6 oz. of fish in total per week.[26]

So, I say to you, if fish isn't good for pregnant women or small children, then I can't see why it should be good for us!

FARMED FISH AND WILD FISH

On January 9, 2004, the results of a serious scientific study, led by Professor Ronald A. Hites, were published in *Science*, one of the most-trusted scientific journals in the world.[27] They produced a global outcry.

The researchers had analyzed seven hundred samples of farmed and wild salmon, purchased in forty different places across the world. They came to the conclusion that the samples were so contaminated that salmon ought to be eaten only occasionally. Following their recommendations would mean once or twice a month.

The French Food Safety Agency had to acknowledge that the contamination figures published in this study were practically identical to what it had found for France (though in France there were slightly higher levels of dioxin and slightly lower levels of PCBs), thus confirming the data. On the other hand, it was unable to issue a counteropinion about the contamination of salmon by toxaphene described in the article, a pesticide so toxic that it has been withdrawn from the worldwide market.[28] So everyone started issuing recommendations, in particular and not surprisingly, the British and Canadian institutions. In the United States, the FDA was fiercely critical of the study, pointing out that the samples analyzed were uncooked and that the skin hadn't been taken off. It even stated that removing the skin and grilling the fish would get rid of most of the toxins that accumulate in the fat in the fish.[29] Try telling this to all the salmon sushi and sashimi fans or to those who enjoy grilled-salmon-skin maki.

Finally, the European Parliament asked the European Food Safety Authority (EFSA) to provide its opinion.[30] The opinion released covers fish such as salmon, trout, carp, herring, anchovies, tuna, mackerel, and sardines.[31] Without going into detail about this long opinion, in one of its chapters it states that given the advances in research in this area, the differences between farmed and wild fish have "decreased." Furthermore, this opinion also states that tuna caught in the wild contains the most mercury. As for PCBs, the highest levels are in wild herring from the Baltic and farmed salmon. However, overall this study concluded that as far as consumer safety is concerned, there is no large-scale difference between farmed fish and wild fish.

Once again, our common sense tells us this ought to be correct because what's causing the contamination of seafood is essentially the sea itself. If both farmed and wild fish are living in the ocean, then there's no logical reason why this contamination should vary widely from one fish to another.

SO DOES THIS MEAN NO FISH AT ALL?

Once again, definitely not!

I really enjoy fish. In spite of everything, fish provides us with phosphorus, iodine, fluoride, zinc, copper, selenium, iron, B vitamins, and vitamin D.[32] These are all extremely important for our nutritional balance and to avoid the major degenerative diseases that threaten us, cancer included. I love fish, but I don't eat just any fish.

First, I avoid tuna altogether, because it's especially contaminated and it's also an endangered species. I do the same with swordfish. I give preference to shrimp, hardly contaminated, over spider crabs, which all too often are polluted.[33]

If I'm eating delicious fish from a lake, I try to check exactly where it came from. I always go for lean, saltwater fish, which as a rule are still completely healthy.

Now we've come to understand that although fish is, no doubt, good for our health, polluted fish is highly dangerous. Together we've examined the reasons for the contamination and the dangers for human health.

We've also learned to be more aware of what fish it is, how to select fish more wisely, and how to make sure that we don't absorb carcinogenic substances from it that will contaminate our bodies for years and years to come.

TABLE 3-5
RECOMMENDATIONS FOR WHAT SEAFOOD TO EAT

	Avoid	Eat
Fish	Eels Marlin Red tuna Salmon Swordfish	Anchovies Bass Mackerel Sardines Sea bream Sole
Crustaceans and shellfish	Spider crabs	Cockles Shrimp

With senseless madness, as if completely oblivious to all the warning signs, we've been polluting our seas over the years, and today they're throwing our pollution back in our faces! So let's try to behave sensibly and work out how to stop ruining our environment. Someday, red tuna and swordfish may become edible once more, even for our grandchildren.

As we wait for this day to come, let's take good care of our health and let's make the right choices. With the "real anticancer advice" in the final chapter, we'll look at what these choices are in greater detail.

Chapter 4

....

Red Meat

LET'S STOP DEMONIZING IT

....

SHOULD WE EAT MEAT OR NOT?

If there's one topic that sparks debate, it's red meat. The health scares that have been associated with meat in recent years, and the way we feel about its quality, its origins, and the conditions in which the animals have been raised, do little to reassure us. It seems that we may have legitimate concerns.

As a matter of fact, we're eating less and less red meat (beef, veal, lamb, and pork). In France, the average consumption has dropped from 1.8 oz. (52 g) per day per person in 2004 to 1.6 oz. (46 g) per day in

---

FOOD COMMODITIES AS MEASURED BY
THE U.S. DEPARTMENT OF AGRICULTURE

The USDA's Economic Research Service (ERS) provides various types of data about food consumption. The ERS Food Availability Per Capita, calculated every year, enables us to measure changes in per capita consumption of major food commodities. The ERS also provides estimates of dietary and nutritional intakes in relation to official dietary guidelines. As for the Total Diet Study, sometimes called the Market Basket Study, it allows us to measure nutrient and contaminant levels for different categories of food commodities.

2007, and in the United States, from 4.8 oz. (137 g) per day per person on average in 2005 to 4.6 oz (131 g) per day in 2009.[1]

This trend started many years ago and clearly continues today. The change in this behavior has been spurred on in recent years by the "mad cow" crisis and the start of the spongiform encephalopathy epidemic that followed. Fortunately, this disastrous health crisis was a real wake-up call for consumers and, more importantly, for the producers and agencies responsible for ensuring that the food we eat is safe. This has resulted in a return to methods of breeding, processing, and distributing meat that promise us greater safety. And yet despite these actions, a recent—mostly unwarranted—attack on red meat has undermined our sense that we can eat it safely, including some experts who say that eating red meat might significantly increase our risk of colon cancer.[2]

So let's look at the figures. By synthesizing the results from seven studies published between 1990 and 2004, six of which showed no serious statistical link between eating red meat and the risk of colon cancer and one, dating from 1994, which claimed the opposite, researchers reached the conclusion that eating red meat frequently increased the risk of colon cancer by 43% compared with eating meat only infrequently.[3] That conclusion dealt with the frequency of consumption. Then, unperturbed by their manipulation of the data, these researchers looked at what happened based on the amount of meat eaten. Once again, they took three studies, of which two had "negative" findings (that is, the results showed no link between the amount of red meat eaten and the risk of colon cancer). By combining these two negative studies with a third study with positive findings (but only for women, not for men), they reached the conclusion that eating 3.5 oz. (100 g) of red meat per day on average would increase our risk of colon cancer by 29%.[4]

If this were true, we'd all have colon cancer! Who'd be able to escape it? Strict vegetarians perhaps? But, in fact, not even them. Further on, we'll see that even vegetarians aren't safe from cancer.

So what should we believe? How can this be possible? If we eat a few slices of ham and five or six small portions of meat a week, is our likelihood of getting colon cancer really that much greater?

Obviously it isn't.

However, rest assured, we're not going to say that, on the one hand, fish may be toxic but that, on the other, as far as meat is concerned, everything is fine. No, definitely not. So let's deal with the different aspects of this huge problem one by one as we try to understand what's going on.

How do we explain that some researchers have reached these conclusions, and why do we believe these conclusions are incorrect?

LET'S START OFF BY BRIEFLY DISCUSSING THESE STUDIES

The total group of studies done includes both case-control and cohort studies (see page 16). As we demonstrated earlier, case-control studies are far less reliable, and since there are more than enough reliable and very extensive cohort studies available for the "red meat–colon cancer" connection, I suggest that we go straight to analyzing them.

One of the best known is the Nurses' Health Study (NHS), a cohort study of almost ninety thousand American female nurses who began being monitored in 1980. In a preliminary report (relying on preliminary reports is never a good idea), written in 1990, with scarcely ten years to take stock, the scientists in charge of the study claimed that women who ate meat every day multiplied their risk of colon cancer by a factor of about 2.5 (again this is women only).[5]

However, after the same cohort of female nurses was studied for a slightly longer period, the final report published in 2004 showed that this increase in risk was a mistake.[6] Whether these women ate red meat *at least three times a month* or *five times or more a week* bore no influence whatsoever on their risk of getting colon cancer.

We're going to look at five further studies in succession, but I'll tell you right now, the results are going to be similar. So for those of you who don't want to bother with such details, you can skip straight to page 57.

The Health Professionals Follow-up Study (HPFS) was a second very extensive cohort study, and it involved just over forty-six thousand men working in the health sector who agreed to be monitored from 1986 on. Here again, the final 2004 report showed that eating red meat frequently—once again, the comparison was between those who eat it *less than three times a month* and those who eat it *five times or more a week*—doesn't in any way increase the risk of getting colon cancer.[7]

The third cohort study was set up in the Netherlands in 1986 and included 120,852 men and women who were then between fifty-five and sixty-nine years old. Those in charge of the investigation confirmed in their final report that there was no connection between eating red meat and the risk of colon cancer (this time it wasn't about how often they ate it but the total amount eaten per day).[8]

The fourth study took place in Finland with a cohort of 9,990 men and women between fifteen and ninety-nine years old and monitored since 1972. It too concluded that there's no link with colon cancer.[9] (However, this study did expose a trend showing that women *who eat fried meat* increase their risk of breast cancer. It's difficult, however, to work out exactly what's due to the meat and what's due to the frying, which we'll take a look at later.)

The fifth study was Norwegian, and it tracked just over fifty thousand people for 11.4 years. This study concluded that *the frequency of consumption of meat in general, of meat-based stews, of roasts, and meatballs was in no way associated with an increase in the risk of colon cancer.*[10]

Lastly, the final and most important cohort study is the European Prospective Investigation into Cancer and Nutrition (EPIC). It looked at 478,040 men and women recruited between 1992 and 1998 from ten European countries, and monitored them on average for five years. In their final report, published in June 2005, the authors showed that there's no definite proof that eating red meat (studied here in terms of daily amounts) increases the risk of colorectal cancer.[11]

This amounts to a lot of serious, important international studies that refute a link between red meat and colon cancer.

Another way of ascertaining whether such a connection exists is to see what happens with vegetarians. Five prospective studies have sought to do this either by comparing vegetarians before and after they became vegetarians, or by comparing vegetarians with "equivalent" non-vegetarian control groups. Two of these studied California Seventh-Day Adventists, followers of a religion that demands that they adhere to a strict vegetarian diet and don't touch a drop of alcohol. Two other studies were British, and the fifth one was German. These five groups included seventy-six thousand volunteers in total. Although the strict vegetarians did indeed have fewer heart attacks, their risk of dying from colon cancer turned out to be absolutely the same as for the non-vegetarians.[12]

Now you know as much as the experts about what these scientific studies have to say on this matter: it's evident that there's no greater risk. Sometimes, though, people still carry on as if these studies said the very opposite. That's fine, and as my daughters would say, we should carry on "as if" the studies are true, and take an even closer look at things.

WE DON'T ALL EAT THE SAME MEAT

When we talk about meat, the French and the Americans are not talking about the same thing. Take 3 ½ oz. (100 g) of fillet steak. The French meat[13] contains 150 calories and the American,[14] 300 calories. French beefsteak is 28% protein,[15] whereas in the United States the same product has only 16% protein.[16] And as for lipids, the fats, it's the reverse. French beefsteak contains 4% lipids,[17] while "made in USA" steak has 24.9%,[18] six times more. This makes all the difference!

When we're eating meat, we're in fact eating something quite different on the two sides of the Atlantic. That's the first point. Imagine that it's the lipids in the meat that are harmful. Then the results recorded from people eating 3.5 oz. (100 g) of American meat full of calories and fat would bear no resemblance at all to the results that would have been recorded if the study had been carried out in France.

The second problem concerns the studies that we've looked at which compared the risk of colon cancer based on the how often red meat was eaten every week. When the French enjoy a meal with red meat, do they eat the same amount as their American friends? Once again, far from it. As we said earlier, a French person eats on average a little under 1.8 oz. (50 g) of red meat per day,[19] whereas an American eats 4.6 oz. (131 g) per day.[20]

That's almost three times as much. We eat very different portion sizes. The French eat less meat per portion, and the meat contains less fat and calories.

And we haven't finished!

TABLE 4-1

DIFFERENCE IN THE NUTRITIONAL COMPOSITION IN MEAT
FROM FRANCE[21] AND THE UNITED STATES[22]

	Cut	Country	Energy (kcal)	Proteins (g)	Lipids (g)	Carbohydrates (g)	MUFAs (g)	PUFAs (g)	Cholesterol (mg)
Beef	Beef steak	United States	295	17	25	10	11	1	70
		France	148	28	4	2	2	1	55
	Roast	United States	297	17	25	10	11	1	70
		France	134	28	2	0.6	0.7	0.3	50
Pork	Chop	United States	282	16	24	9	11	2	81
		France	175	19	11	4	5	1	54
Veal	Shoulder (shank)	United States	132	19	5	2	2	0.4	82
		France	134	19	7	3	3	0.3	81
Chicken	Breast	United States	114	23	2	0.4	0.4	0.4	58
		France	118	22	3	0.8	1	0.6	61
	Drumstick	United States	187	18	12	3	5	3	83
		France	231	26	14	4	6	3	122

Note: MUFAs, monounsaturated fatty acids; PUFAs, polyunsaturated fatty acids.

TABLE 4-2

PORTION SIZE IN FRANCE[23] AND IN THE UNITED STATES[24, 25]

Country	Average portion size per day
France	Meat: 1.8 oz. (49.7 g) Poultry and game: 1.1 oz. (31.9 g)
United States	Meat: 4.6 oz. (131 g) Poultry: 3.0 oz. (86 g)

Do we cook our meat the same way? Once again, we do things quite differently. Americans prefer to grill or barbecue meat. Cooking meat this way turns the surface of the meat black, which produces highly carcinogenic polycyclic hydrocarbons. Another disadvantage is that, traditionally, Americans cook their meat medium to well done, which causes a similar increase in carcinogens.

The French, however, put a little fat in the bottom of a frying pan, which comes between the meat and the broiling metal so that the meat gets cooked more gently, resulting in fewer carcinogenic carbons on the meat's surface, and they eat their meat far less well done. As consumer surveys show, the French also often eat their meat raw, either as tartare or as carpaccio. In addition, they eat meat that has been simmered (in casseroles, stews, etc.), often removing the fat from the cooking juices. As you can see, the French cook in far more varied ways and often in healthier ways as far as cancer is concerned.

Lastly and perhaps most importantly, as we discussed in our introduction, when we eat meat, we never eat it on its own. When you sit down to eat, don't you think that what's served along with your beefsteak is likely to alter the biological and metabolic effects of the various elements of food that you're about to swallow? Of course it does. I'll give you an example.

A recent French study showed that 20% of the French population eats more than 2.5 oz. (70 g) of red meat per day—that is, over 17 oz. (500 g) per week (and, conversely, 56% of the population eats less than 1.6 oz. (45 g) per day.[26] The first are very big red-meat eaters, and as with any excess, this eating habit can quite possibly increase the risk of cancer. Why?

Look around you carefully: watch these great meat eaters, and straightaway you'll see that they amass harmful habits that might well promote certain cancers. And, unfortunately, none of the studies that focused on meat have taken account of this fact. Fiber intake for major red-meat consumers is generally paltry, although it's very important for digestion. These people don't tend to hanker after steamed or raw vegetables, often preferring a large plate of fries, full of saturated fatty acids and therefore unhealthy. Cereals seldom appear in their diet, and their consumption of fruit, with its powerful antioxidant effect, falls below recommended daily guidelines.

As we'll see time and again in this book, all long-term excess should be outlawed. In saying this, we're simply recommending our eating habits from yesteryear, which weren't so bad after all. Taking things to an extreme is never good, with the exception of living it up from time to time. So if eating a grilled rib of beef once in a while gives you pleasure, go ahead! Otherwise, be sensible.

As we'll see in the last chapter, titled "Anticancer Advice," a practical approach when you're eating meat is to check where the meat comes from and choose naturally grass-fed, lean meat. If you're pan-frying it, don't overdo it. Avoid grilling your meat, and try other ways of cooking it too. Remove the fat from your meat juices and stocks. Eat other healthy foods with your meat, which we'll look at later.

Since the beginning of time, humans have always eaten meat. Starting out, the first humans were hunter-gatherers for thousands of years. They lived on what they could forage (in general, fruit, berries, and plants) and hunt. They didn't grow crops or rear animals. Nevertheless, when we examine human remains dating from that time, we see that they had no more cancers than we do now, even at the same age, although their life expectancy was far shorter than ours, due to many reasons other than cancer. It didn't stop these people from discovering fire, bronze, the wheel, the plow, and so on, and from developing great civilizations.

But let's get back to the present day.

HOW TRADITIONAL WAYS CAN
HELP WITH PREVENTION

There's another point I'd like to highlight about red meat, one that can really help protect against cancer. Ask yourself what constituents of meat are heavily emphasized as playing a harmful role in cancer.

Several hypotheses have been put forward, but the most interesting one by far points the blame at the hemoglobin found in the blood in red meat. Hemoglobin, which gives blood (the red blood cells, in fact) its red color, transports oxygen from the lungs, where the blood is oxygenated, toward the peripheral tissues, which require oxygen in order to ensure the necessary combustion for cell metabolism. We looked at this process in the second chapter.

Hemoglobin has three components: the organic molecule heme, the protein chain globin, and an iron molecule. We now know that heme encourages the formation of N-nitroso compounds, which are potentially very toxic and carcinogenic.[27] As for the iron, it might make highly reactive free radicals appear, which are likely to damage our DNA and thereby induce carcinogenic mutation.[28] Moreover, iron stimulates the secretion of pro-inflammatory substances[29] and encourages the production of blood vessels, which are then able to supply more fresh blood to a potential tumor intent on growing.

One way of avoiding this risk may be to follow the ancient Muslim and Jewish practices of draining the blood from meat before cooking it. This is in fact exactly what great chefs do when they leave cooked meat to rest before serving it. After the thermal shock of cooking, the meat relaxes, and as it does so, the blood is gradually released. You should add this practice to your anticancer diet.

This theory about the role hemoglobin plays in the blood of red meat and it being involved in the development of certain cancers has been comprehensively demonstrated in many animals.[30, 31] It seems the most probable hypothesis in light of the many scientific articles I've read on the subject, and thus the most likely theory.

However, and this is an important point as we compile our anticancer advice, a certain practice may completely inhibit this pro-carcinogenic effect, one that has been thoroughly proved in animals: taking a calcium tablet after meals. According to a team of French researchers, this simple act may counteract the blood's carcinogenic effect on the intestinal mucosa.[32] So if you don't want to drain the blood from your meat, you could swallow a calcium pill.

AND WHAT ABOUT WHITE MEAT AND POULTRY?

Less fatty, especially if you remove the skin, and containing less hemoglobin, white meat and poultry (pork, turkey, chicken) are not mentioned as possible cancer promoters in any studies.[33] I won't analyze them here. They're neutral as far as the risk of cancer is concerned. You can eat as much as you like of them.

IN THIS CHAPTER, we've taken a critical perspective toward people who are willing to mix up all kinds of ideas in order to prove what they want to think or believe. The only truth is that which has been proved independently and repeatedly by science. Implausible combinations of studies with negative results and those that are positive, a mixture of different products that are neither identical nor comparable, the disregard of common sense and traditions that have accompanied humankind in harmonious development—all these irregularities, as far as we're concerned, don't offer us guidance for formulating eating habits.

Chapter 5

·················

Do Dairy Products and Eggs Help Prevent Cancer?

··

Discussing the links between dairy products and cancer is not the easiest undertaking.

There are several reasons. First, dairy products encompass a multitude of different foods ranging from fresh milk, which can be whole, low fat, or fat free, to cheeses, which can have widely differing effects depending on the extent to which they've been fermented. Yogurts can also be made with many different cultures (bacillus), so their impact on our health can be just as variable. The same goes for products made with raw milk (that is, with its natural enzymes) versus pasteurized milk (into which producers usually add certain microorganisms).

As we'll see, there is also a great genetic inequality between those who can "digest" milk and those who cannot, often connected to the geographic region from which their ancestors came. Lastly, to explain where dairy products stand in our anticancer diet, we'll need to introduce two new concepts: prebiotics and probiotics.

Ever since humans learned to milk mammals, milk and milk products have helped us develop, helped our children grow, and kept us healthy. Why not stop here? Can't we simply assume that since milk seems good for our children, then surely it ought to be equally good for the rest of us? Unfortunately, it really isn't possible to simplify things this way.

Let's start by explaining the three tools that we're going to need to understand the connections between dairy and cancer risks. Two of them, prebiotics and probiotics, you may have heard talked about in the media, though I've noticed that they get confused the majority of the time. The third tool is an enzyme, galactosidase, which some of us have in our gut and is the reason why milk is not necessarily good for all adults.

LET'S START WITH PREBIOTICS AND PROBIOTICS

Probiotics are living bacteria we ingest that are capable of breaking down certain dangerous compounds. They detoxify a lot of the harmful material in our intestines,[1] which was either present in our food or produced by digestion. In people who are lactose intolerant, probiotics improve their digestion and absorption of lactose.[2] Probiotics stimulate the immune system and can prevent the mutation of DNA and therefore cancer. Finally, probiotics tend to destroy the microorganisms, sometimes found in the intestinal flora, that are likely to produce carcinogenic substances.[3] Still, while probiotics are good for our health, they aren't all equally good at preventing cancer.

Some foods (sunchokes, garlic, bananas, chicory, onions, barley, asparagus, etc.) help speed up digestion because they contain biocompounds (fiber, oligosaccharides, etc.) that our bowels cannot digest. These are prebiotics. As soon as they reach the bowels, they become the preferred target for a fermentation process associated with the bacteria found there, and they then stimulate the production of nonpathogenic bacteria (probiotics).[4] Thanks to this fermentation, a large amount of glutathione S-transferase, an enzyme we've already discussed, is produced locally in the colon. If there's any enzyme capable of detoxifying most carcinogenic products, it is glutathione S-transferase.[5] Another compound we looked at in chapter 2, butyrate, is also produced by this fermentation process. Butyrate is a powerful inhibitor of the genotoxic activity (that is, toxic for genes) of nitrosamines and hydrogen peroxide, two fearsome carcinogenic compounds.[6] Both prebiotics and probiotics are fundamental to preventing colon cancer, especially if cleverly combined,[7] in which case they are called "symbiotics."

GALACTOSIDASE, A PROTECTIVE ENZYME

Another important enzyme, galactosidase, is produced (if indeed it is produced, and we'll come back to this question later) in the first part of our intestines.[8] This enzyme is capable of digesting lactose, which is a double sugar or "disaccharide" found in milk and some milk products (see Table 5-1).

When galactosidase is present, the lactose is divided into two simple sugars: glucose and galactose, which are then absorbed by the intestines. If there is insufficient galactosidase, or if there is none at all, the lactose is not digested. Undigested lactose lingers in the colon, where the microbial flora turns it into lactic acid.[9] This acid irritates and eventually inflames the intestinal cells, producing "oxidative stress." In other words, it triggers the appearance of oxygen radicals, which corrode the DNA and make it susceptible to changes to the genetic code and could therefore, at least theoretically, cause a cancerous cell to appear.

TABLE 5-1

LACTOSE CONTENT OF CERTAIN DAIRY PRODUCTS[10]

Dairy product	Serving size	Lactose content	Lactose Percentage
Milk, regular	8 oz.	.4 oz.	4.80%
Milk, skim	8 oz.	.5 oz.	5.20%
Yogurt, plain, regular	7 oz.	.3 oz.	4.50%
Yogurt, plain, low fat	7 oz.	.4 oz.	6.00%
Cheddar cheese	1 oz.	.0007 oz.	.07%
Cottage cheese	1 oz.	.003 oz.	.33%
Butter	1 tsp.	.001 oz.	.51%
Ice cream	2 oz.	.1 oz.	6.00%

DIGESTING MILK

Galactosidase is almost always found in children, but in puberty it tends to disappear in most of us.[11] From a health perspective, milk is important because it contains calcium and vitamin D, two substances that are vital for our bodies' growth and for the prevention of rickets, a serious illness. However, there's another way to get vitamin D, a vitamin that enables us to retain calcium in our bodies, particularly in our bones. When our is skin exposed to sunlight, it too produces vitamin D. In the history of human evolution, as more populations became naturally exposed to the sun because of their geographic location, the more the sun stimulated their skin to produce the amount of vitamin D they needed, and the less dependent they became on milk for vitamin D. These populations therefore gradually stopped producing galactosidase and drank less and less milk since they found it hard to digest. This was what happened to populations in the southern part of the Northern Hemisphere. Conversely, with far less opportunity for exposure to sunlight, the populations living in the northern part transmitted their galactosidase from generation to generation very actively, because without it they would have all succumbed to rickets. We see this happening today: 80% of Belgians have active galactosidase; of people living around the Mediterranean, 25% to 50% have it; and barely 20% of Africans do (see Table 5-2).[12] These statistics are why we have to take ethnicity into account when talking about dairy products. They also show why we must not try to go against dietary traditions and practices embedded in each local region.

DAIRY PRODUCTS AND THE RISK OF CANCER

What do the countless studies recommend regarding dairy products and preventing cancer? A fairly common finding is that eating lots of dairy products significantly increases the risk of prostate cancer.[13] Since this is by far the most common type of cancer in men,[14] it seems rather pointless to further increase one's risk.

TABLE 5-2

LACTOSE INTOLERANCE ACROSS THE WORLD:
THE NORTH-SOUTH GRADIENT[15]

	Proportion with lactose intolerance
Asians	95–100%
American Indians	80–100%
Africans and African Americans	60–80%
Ashkenazi Jews	60–80%
Hispanics	50–80%
Southern Indians	60–70%
Northern Indians	20–30%
Central Europeans	9–23%
White Americans	6–22%
Northern Europeans	2–15%

The same goes for increasing calcium intake from dairy products (however, not for non-dietary calcium, that is, calcium tablets). A man with a total daily calcium intake of .07 oz. (2 g) from dairy products has an almost 30% higher risk of getting prostate cancer than a man who consumes less than .03 oz. (1 g) a day.[16]

Does this mean that adults should avoid dairy products altogether? Actually, no, because they might prevent colon cancers. However, not all studies agree on this point. Given the great variations between dairy products in different countries as well as the variations among individuals in their ability to digest milk, it is quite difficult to reach a general conclusion.

The E3N-EPIC study, an important study published at the end of 2005, deserves to be mentioned. It compared two populations: 172 patients with colon cancer and 67,312 control subjects who did not suffer from any type of cancer. The participants were questioned about their eating habits, and in particular about the dairy products they ate. Overall, the researchers were unable to show any clear, conclusive difference: drinking milk is not clearly related to a reduced risk of colon

TABLE 5-3

CALCIUM CONTENT IN DAIRY PRODUCTS[17]

Dairy products	Serving size	Calcium content (mg)	Number of Calories
Milk, 1% low fat	8 oz.	300	102
Milk, 2% low fat	8 oz.	297	121
Milk, skim	8 oz.	302	86
Milk, whole	8 oz.	291	150
Yogurt, plain, whole milk	8 oz.	274	139
Yogurt, plain, low fat	8 oz.	400	130
American cheese	1 oz.	150	110
Cheddar cheese	1 oz.	204	114
Cheddar cheese, 1% low fat	½ cup	69	82
Cream cheese	1 oz. or 2 tbsp.	23	99
Mozzarella cheese	1 oz.	147	80
Parmesan cheese, grated	2 tbsp.	138	46
Swiss cheese	1 oz.	272	107

cancer, although it could lower the risk of developing (benign) intestinal polyps, which are often precursors for cancers.[18]

However—and this is where it gets complicated—some American studies showed that individuals who drink a lot of milk (almost 7 oz. (200 mL) to 10 oz. (300 mL) a day) benefited from a modest (around 10%) reduction in their risk of colon cancer, compared to those who drink hardly any milk (less than 2 oz. (70 mL) a day). Keep in mind, though, that the risk was lower only for cancers in the distal (lower) part of the colon.[19]

Last, let's take a careful look at Table 5-4. Although there are no data available for the United States, the table shows that there is actually no correlation between a nation's higher dairy consumption and lower incidence of colon cancer. For example, Switzerland, which in our table has the largest average dairy-product consumption per inhabitant, has a higher mortality rate for colorectal cancer than does Italy (where dairy-product consumption is 26% lower per inhabitant per year) or Japan (67% lower).

So what should we do? Whenever we're faced such perplexing situations, I think we should try to ask the question the other way around. Do we actually need to eat lots of dairy products?

There's no question that children need dairy products to grow. It is really important that they are not deprived of them, especially since at their age prostate problems aren't an issue.

But do adults need dairy products? Women do, particularly after menopause. Once women have stopped secreting hormones, their natural tendency to develop osteoporosis, a condition involving thinning of the bones caused by bone demineralization, is accentuated. So women, in particular those who are pregnant, breastfeeding, menopausal, or premenopausal (just before menopause), need lots of calcium and vitamin D and could benefit from eating dairy products or taking calcium and vitamin D supplements. Here again, there's no prostate problem because, of course, women don't have prostates.

But what about men? I believe that men should be very careful with dairy products. Unless your family and the people in the area you come from have done otherwise since time immemorial, it is best to

TABLE 5-4

**THE RELATIONSHIP BETWEEN EATING DAIRY PRODUCTS
AND COLON CANCER[20]**

Country	Dairy product consumption (kg/year)	Low lactasic activity (%)	Mortality from colorectal cancer (per 100,000 inhabitants)	
			Men	Women
Switzerland	133	10	17.8	10.5
Canada	122	6	16.9	11.2
France	116	37	17.4	10.1
Australia	110	6	20.2	13.7
Spain	109	23	14.6	9.4
Germany	102	15	21.3	15.1
Italy	98	50	15.3	9.9
Japan	43	93	15.7	9.8
United States	n/a	15	16.5	11.2

Note: n/a, not available.

**3 DAIRY PRODUCTS PER DAY IS EQUIVALENT
TO ANY OF THE FOLLOWING:**

- 1 cup of milk (choose fat-free or low-fat milk), 1 regular container of yogurt (8 oz.), 1 cup of rice pudding made with milk
- ½ cup of ricotta cheese, 2 slices of Swiss cheese (¾ oz. each), 1 cup of frozen yogurt
- 1 cup of cottage cheese, 2 oz. of Gouda cheese, 1 cup of chocolate milk (choose fat-free or low-fat milk)
- 1 cup of calcium-fortified soymilk, 1 cup of chocolate pudding (made with whole milk), ⅓ cup of shredded cheddar cheese

---

avoid milk and instead to get your calcium from cheese, which naturally has a far higher calcium content. Yogurts provide the most suitable probiotics for men. However, the yogurt absolutely must contain two strains of bacteria proved to be excellent for men: *Lactobacillus bulgaricus* and *Streptococcus thermophilus*.[21] These strains usually remain alive until the very last day of their use-by date. If men do eat lots of dairy products, they should eat them with large amounts of prebiotics (why not try a nice banana smoothie?) to speed up their digestion. Once they've finished digesting, they should then have what is called a "scavenger" meal—that is, a meal high in antioxidants that will repair the damage that might have been produced in the DNA of their prostate cells, for example, a meal with lots of fruits and vegetables, especially tomatoes and pomegranate juice, all, of course, with plenty of green tea.

EGGS

Before we finish this chapter, a quick word about eggs. Nutritionally, eggs are extremely healthy, and there is no serious study showing a possible link with the risk of cancer.[22] Let's rank eggs together with other foods that are cancer neutral. This means eggs are recommended, and if you have no cholesterol problems, you can eat as many as you like.

Chapter 6

....

Fruits and Vegetables

BENEFITS BUT NO CERTAINTIES

....

Let's move on to talk about produce now. For some years there has
been an unprecedented campaign promoting the theme that fruits
and vegetables protect you from cancer. The U.S. Department of Agriculture's Choose My Plate program, for example, following the 2010
Dietary Guidelines for Americans, says on its website that you should
"make half your plate fruits and vegetables."[1] Stepping into the fray, the
food-processing industry has come up with dozens of produce-based
products, latching onto this new "eat well to be healthy" trend, singing
ever louder the praises of fruits and veggies and their famous antioxidant properties.

So are fruits and vegetables our panacea? Do they really protect
us from cancer? In its 2007 report, the highly reputable World Cancer Research Fund, while suggesting that fruits and vegetables have
some involvement in preventing cancer (see Table 6-1), ends its chapter about the preventive impact of fruits and vegetables on cancer by
saying, "Findings from cohort studies conducted since the mid-1990s
have made the overall evidence that vegetables, or fruits, protect against
cancers, somewhat less impressive."[2]

Well, well! To avoid cancer, we are told we need to stuff ourselves

TABLE 6-1

**SUMMARY OF THE WORLD CANCER RESEARCH FUND'S
CONCLUSIONS ABOUT THE LINK BETWEEN EATING FRUITS
AND VEGETABLES AND GETTING CANCER**

Factor	Decreases risk of cancer of the	Level of proof
Non-starchy vegetables	Mouth, pharynx, larynx, esophagus, stomach	Probable
Fruits	Mouth, pharynx, larynx, esophagus, stomach, lung	Probable
Foods containing carotenoids	Mouth, pharynx, larynx, lung	Probable
Foods containing beta-carotene	Esophagus	Probable
Foods containing lycopene	Prostate	Probable

with fruits and vegetables every day, without even knowing which ones, and yet the world's leading experts state that it's impossible to conclude irrefutably that doing so is truly beneficial.

So who should we believe? Why is there so much uncertainty? To my mind, the reason is simple. Fruits and vegetables contain a little over a hundred thousand phytocompounds, which may be fiber, micronutrients, microconstituents, and many other things.

Much depends on how we eat the produce: raw or cooked, crushed or whole, peeled or with the skin on, organic or with pesticide residues. It may also depend on whether we eat it alone or as an accompaniment to other foods (for example, green beans with a steak), at what time of the day we eat it, whether we are male or female, adult or child. There is such enormous variability and terrifying complexity here, more so than for the other types of food we've looked at, that unless specifically trained to deal with these nutritional issues, most of us wouldn't know where to start or how to create an outline about the ways we should be eating fruits and vegetables and which particular ones.

Once again, we've tried to simplify the information for you, so that we can deduce some easy rules that we'll give you later in the anticancer advice chapter of this book (see page 151). However, some of you might first like to learn a little about what fruits and vegetables have to offer. Some basic information will help you better understand the scientific and nutritional specifics involved here.

WHAT'S THE DIFFERENCE BETWEEN MICRONUTRIENTS AND MICROCONSTITUENTS?

The first, micronutrients, are nutrients that the body needs in small quantities in order for it to function properly and remain healthy. We must ingest these micronutrients from our food and drink because our bodies cannot make them. This is the case, for example, with vitamins and minerals.

Microconstituents, on the other hand, are chemical compounds found in tiny quantities in foods. The human body does not absolutely need them to function properly. They include, for example, certain antioxidants, such as polyphenols and anthocyanins. Both types of elements can play a key role in the prevention of cancers. We'll return to this shortly.

Why are antioxidants, thoroughly bound up with produce, so important? To oversimplify, it is because of the damage created when each of the millions of billions of cells in our body engages in cell respiration—the releasing of energy from food—and as a result produces very toxic free radicals. As we saw earlier, each day the DNA in each of our cells undergoes almost ten thousand mutations.

Our exposure to the sun and oxygen—necessary for our survival—is the reason why our cells constantly form these free radicals, which are strongly reactive with our cell components and, in particular, with our DNA and thus the genes that are inscribed on it. These corrosive free radicals are capable of damaging the makeup of our cells, the DNA and the proteins, in a fraction of a second. These radicals are very toxic for our health, and they're responsible for cell aging and degeneration. This fact creates a double-edged sword since without oxygen it's impossible for us to produce the energy that our cells must have to grow, renew themselves, and survive.[3]

TABLE 6-2

THE TOP ANTIOXIDANT-RICH FRUITS AND VEGETABLES

Fruit		Vegetables	
Name	Antioxidant score (ORAC/100 g)	Name	Antioxidant score (ORAC/100 g)
Prunes	5,770	Kale	1,770
Raisins	2,830	Spinach	1,260
Blueberries	2,400	Brussels sprouts	980
Blackberries	2,036	Alfalfa sprouts	930
Strawberries	1,540	Broccoli	890
Raspberries	1,220	Beets	840
Plums	949	Red peppers	710
Oranges	750	Onions	450
Red grapes	739	Corn	400
Cherries	670	Eggplant	390
Kiwi	602		
Pink grapefruit	483		

Note: ORAC, oxygen radical absorption capacity.

Fortunately, the human machine is particularly well constructed and has developed a fantastic strategy to cope with this enemy, the free radicals that our cells produce by "respiration" (metabolism). The body has a powerful antioxidant defense system that continuously controls the free radicals' oxidative damage, which we sometimes call "oxidative stress." This system works as a sort of rustproof paint with which our bodies brush our cells, the oxidative damage being similar to the rust that destroys and ages everything metal, especially as that is due to none other than the oxidation of iron by oxygen.

In our bodies, antioxidants such as vitamin C, vitamin E, and lycopene, to mention just three, work to oppose the free radicals.[4] Usually, enzymes then take over and finish repairing the damage within the cells to prevent them from transforming into malignant cells. Ultimately, the system is very well developed, but it does require an effective synergy between the antioxidants and the enzymes.

The antioxidant effect can occur directly or indirectly. Certain trace elements found in our food (such as zinc, selenium, and manganese) have, for example, direct antioxidant properties, as do vitamins C and E, carotenoids, polyphenols, and even alliaceous compounds (found in garlic and onion). They all have a direct effect on the cell components.

Other elements such as chrome and magnesium act more indirectly. Chrome does so by improving insulin sensitivity, which has an impact on weight and therefore the risk of cancer (see page 137). Another, magnesium, combats the potentially pro-carcinogenic effect of inflammation.[5] As we're reflecting on how to lower our risk through food and drink of getting cancer—no matter how high that risk is—it's important to know that a fundamental principle is not to eat something whenever we feel like it, on the pretext that it has antioxidants. What is important is that we keep to the optimum balance and dosage that are right for us of the different phytocompounds, according to their various antioxidant properties.

COLORS AND THEIR PROTECTIVE PROPERTIES

To make your life simple, I've decided to talk to you about fruits and vegetables according to their color.

Their color? But, you are going to say, didn't you tell us in your introduction that we should be on the lookout for all sorts of crazy things, which sound more or less phony, that we get told about foods and cancer. And now, all of a sudden, you want us to believe you when you tell us that you're going to talk to us about the benefits of fruits and vegetables based on their color?

My answer is yes. This is indeed correct, and the reason is extremely simple. The vast majority of these well-known phytocompounds that can repair our genes, stabilize our DNA, and detoxify carcinogenic substances—these compounds that have antioxidant properties, pro-methylation (see page 37 on the silencing of dangerous genes), or antiproliferative properties, or even contain substances that

TABLE 6-3

**PHYTOCHEMICAL COMPOUNDS FOUND IN FRUITS AND
VEGETABLES ACCORDING TO COLOR[6]**

Color	Phytochemical compounds	Main products
Green	Glucosinolates	Broccoli, cabbage
Orange	Alpha- and beta-carotene	Carrots, mangoes, pumpkins
Red	Lycopene	Tomatoes
Purple	Anthocyanins	Grapes, blackberries, raspberries, cranberries, blueberries
Orange-yellow	Flavonoids	Honeydew melons, peaches, papaya, oranges, tangerines
Green-yellow	Lutein and zeaxanthin	Spinach, corn, avocadoes, melons
White and cream	Allicin and phytoestrogens	Garlic, onions, soy, radishes

can modulate our immune system—are the same as those that give each fruit and vegetable its particular color.

As a general rule, these phytocompounds are the pigments that give our fruits and vegetables their color.

So why not group them together according to their specific virtues for cancer—that is, according to the phytocompounds they contain, and therefore in practice, their color? Each color, in fact, has its pluses.

The color green

Glucosinolates are the compounds responsible for the green color and are derivatives of amino acids containing sulfur.[7] They can be transformed into isothiocyanates and indoles. A link has been established between some of these substances and a reduced risk of oral, esophageal, stomach, and lung cancer.[8] Their anticarcinogenic effect comes from the activation of enzymes (see page 37) that are involved in the detoxification of carcinogenic agents, as well as from the inhibition of enzymes that modify the metabolism of steroidal hormones (which

TABLE 6-4

**GREEN FRUITS AND VEGETABLES WITH
THE MOST INDOLE COMPOUNDS[9]**

Best sources of indole in green fruits and vegetables		
Broccoli	Brussels sprouts	Rutabaga
Cauliflower	Kale	Watercress
Cabbage	Chinese cabbage	Turnips

as you know are carcinogenic) and from the protection against oxidative damage.[10]

Indole, which is particularly found in cabbage, could equally help prevent cancer of the colon and stomach, along with cancers of the lung, esophagus, rectum, and bladder.[11]

In a 2006 study, men who ate vegetables from the cabbage family at least twice a week saw their risk of getting pancreatic cancer drop by almost 40%.[12] Moreover, green leafy vegetables contain a high level of folic acid and chlorophyll.[13] Folic acid protects against pancreatic cancer.[14] Chlorophyll has a structure almost identical to the hemoglobin found in our red blood cells, which we saw was probably responsible for the potentially carcinogenic effect of consuming too much animal blood (blood sausage, meat that has not rested or had its blood drained off etc.). Chlorophyll seems to have properties that detoxify the hemoglobin.[15] To secure the benefits of plant photosynthesis from the presence of carbon dioxide and sunlight, you should always consume a chlorophyll-containing food at the same time you eat meat, especially in the evening. This has been shown to be beneficial in several animal studies.[16, 17] Remember, then, to eat green vegetables with meat.

The color orange

Orange fruits and vegetables are full of carotenoids (alpha- and beta-carotenes), which give them their color.

TABLE 6-5

**ORANGE FRUITS AND VEGETABLES
WITH THE MOST BETA-CAROTENE[18]**

Best sources of beta-carotene in orange fruits and vegetables	
Mangoes	Squash
Carrots	Peaches
Sweet potatoes	Pumpkins
Apricots	

There are between forty and fifty carotenoids in our diet. Potentially they can be transformed into vitamin A, which plays a role in cell differentiation, in modulation of the immune system, in regulation of cell proliferation, and in the synthesis of hormones. They are powerful antioxidants[19] and are better absorbed if the fruit or vegetable is cooked beforehand, eaten puréed, or prepared with some oil added since they're liposoluble compounds.[20]

Carotenoids protect from oral, lung, and esophageal cancers.[21] They might play a role in preventing cervical cancer owing to their immunological effects on the human papillomavirus (HPV)[22] that causes this disease. They might also help prevent prostate cancer. However, be careful, as they might be dangerous if you are a smoker.

The color orange-yellow

In certain fruits and vegetables, flavonoids along with beta-cryptoxanthin are responsible for their light-orange-verging-on-yellow color.

Flavonoids have antiviral, anti-inflammatory, and antioxidant properties. They inhibit lipid peroxidation, which is highly carcinogenic, and they trap free radicals.

Flavonoids, which are polyphenols, are able to accelerate the metabolism of carcinogenic substances.[23] One of these flavonoids, quercetin—found in abundance in lovage and hot chili peppers, as well as in capers and cocoa—is an inhibitor of cytochromes and phase

TABLE 6-6

**ORANGE-YELLOW FRUITS AND VEGETABLES CONTAINING
THE MOST BIOFLAVONOIDS[24]**

Best sources of bioflavonoids in orange-yellow fruits and vegetables		
Oranges	Apricots	Pears
Grapefruit	Peaches	Pineapples
Lemons	Nectarines	Green grapes
Tangerines	Papaya	Yellow sweet peppers
Clementines		

I enzymes which stimulate the development of cancers (see page 38). It has been clearly shown that quercetin can reduce the carcinogenic effect of tobacco.[25]

The color red

The color red in produce is due to lycopene, which also belongs to the carotenoid family and so works as a powerful antioxidant. Furthermore, it's the precursor for other members of the carotenoid family that are found in other foods that we eat and drink.

Unlike the other members in this family of antioxidants, lycopene does not transform into vitamin A.[26] This is important because its activities will be different from those of vitamin A. It plays an important role in intercellular and intracellular communication. We've seen earlier that this communication is at the base of cell reactions to growth factors that stimulate cell proliferation. Tomatoes, notably, contain a lot of lycopene, which definitely prevents prostate cancer, reducing the risk by almost 30%.[27] It might reduce the risk of other cancers, such as oral, esophageal, stomach, and lung cancer.[28]

Products made from fresh tomatoes often contain more lycopene than actual tomatoes.[29] This is because when they are turned into a paste, juice, sauce, or ketchup, the lycopene is more concentrated and in this phytocompound can be better absorbed. Its bioavailability is

TABLE 6-7

RED FRUITS AND VEGETABLES PROVIDING THE MOST
LYCOPENE AND ANTHOCYANINS[30]

Best sources of lycopene in red fruits and vegetables	Best sources of anthocyanins in red fruits and vegetables
Tomato juice	Raspberries
Tomato soup	Strawberries
Fresh tomatoes	Cranberries
Watermelons	Red cabbage
Guava	Red kidney beans
Pink grapefruit	Cherries
	Beets
	Red apples
	Red onions

further improved if eaten with some oil, for example, as in a sauce for pasta. So long live those Italian recipes.

The color purple

Anthocyanins and phenols give fruits and vegetables their purple color. They're also powerful antioxidants, capable of blocking the harmful effects that free radicals produce during cell metabolism.

These anthocyanins are anticarcinogenic substances, and through a pro-apoptotic effect they try to stop cancers from developing,[31] as you read earlier, by stimulating cells with damaged genes to commit suicide.

They also protect us from cancer by acting like a veritable sunscreen. As it happens, these anthocyanins are very effective at absorbing solar ultraviolet radiation, which can potentially cause cancer when we expose our skin to the sun.[32] If you're often out in the sun or have had a skin cancer, you should eat plenty of foods containing anthocyanins.

Studies have shown that anthocyanins could protect us from cancer of the colon by reducing the proliferation of cells in the mucous membrane of the colon,[33] and one of these anthocyanins, delphinidin,

TABLE 6-8

PURPLE FRUITS AND VEGETABLES PROVIDING THE MOST
ANTHOCYANINS AND POLYPHENOLS[34]

Best sources of anthocyanins in purple fruits and vegetables	Best sources of polyphenols in purple fruits and vegetables
Blueberries	Prunes
Red grapes	Grapes
Blackberries	Eggplant
Black currants	Plums
Elderberries	

might protect us from liver cancer.[35] These molecules are able to block receptors for factors that stimulate cell proliferation and, in particular, the receptors for growth factor in epidermal cells (epidermal growth factor receptor, or EGFR).[36]

The color green-yellow

Some produce have a green-yellow color because they contain lutein and zeaxanthin, two pigments that belong to the xanthophylls family, which is itself part of the carotenoid family.[37]

Lutein can arrest the cell cycle, thereby preventing cell division and stimulating damaged cells to commit suicide (apoptosis),[38] which has been demonstrated in cancerous cells taken from patients with leu-

TABLE 6-9

GREEN-YELLOW FRUITS AND VEGETABLES
WITH THE MOST LUTEIN[39]

Best sources of lutein in green-yellow fruits and vegetables	
Kale	Garden peas
Spinach	Honeydew melons
Romaine lettuce	Kiwi
Broccoli	Leafy vegetables (mustard, turnips)

kemia or with skin, liver, or pancreatic cancer.[40] This effect has also been observed in human prostate-cancer cells that have been transplanted into mice.[41]

The color white or cream

There are three sorts of foods in this fruit and vegetable group: soy; radishes, horseradish, and chicory; and, lastly, garlic and onions.

It seems that eating soy—which is high in phytoestrogens—can lower the risk of breast cancer.[42] This effect has been shown several times in studies on humans and appears quite logical. Moreover, this is also the mechanism that in general explains the low incidence of breast cancer in Japanese women, whose average consumption of soy is known to be far greater than that of American or European women[43] (8.8 lb. [4 kg] of tofu per person in Japan, compared with 5.3 oz. [150 g] per person in Europe and the United States in the 1990s).[44] Eating lots of soy might reduce the risk of colorectal cancer for menopausal women,[45] and it might play a role in protecting against the risk of stomach cancer.[46] Only drinking soy milk, however, may reduce the risk for prostate cancer.[47] This effect is the result of saponins and genistein,[48] inhibitors of pro-carcinogenic enzymes (phase I enzymes, see page 38). These compounds might also stop the extension of blood vessels that feed a tumor, thereby depriving the tumor of fresh blood and, thus, killing the cancerous cells.[49]

The second group is composed of radishes, horseradish, and chicory. These foods seem able to significantly lower the risk of stomach cancer, possibly up to 30% to 40%.[50] They're low in calories, so it's good to eat plenty of them.

Finally, the third group includes garlic and onions and their derivatives. These vegetables contain allicin, a powerful antioxidant that is antiviral, anticarcinogenic, and detoxifying.[51] The enzyme alliinase operates on the compound alliin to form allicin. Garlic has to be peeled and crushed for the alliinase inside to be released. If garlic is heated without first being peeled, this enzyme will be inactivated. However, alliinase remains active in garlic that is crushed or diced.[52]

These foods play an extremely important role in reducing the risk of stomach cancer. For people who eat copious amounts of them, that can mean a 40% risk reduction. The same effect may be achieved for the risk of colon cancer.[53] So don't hesitate to use them in everything!

AS WE'VE SEEN, THERE'S A genuine and extremely complex link between eating fruits and vegetables and the risk of a particular cancer. We can say that overall fruits and vegetables are good for preventing cancer. Not only are they good because of the phytocompounds they contain, which may have specific properties regarding the processes that turn cells cancerous, but there are two other equally good reasons for eating them.

They're low-calorie foods. By consuming them you can avoid putting on weight, because your stomach fills up and you feel satisfied. High in sugars and with a relatively low glycemic index, they don't increase your appetite with a rebound effect. They stop you from becoming overweight, which, as we'll see later, appears as an incredible risk factor in the study of cancer.

The second reason is that, as a rule, fruits and vegetables are high in fiber. For a long time now, a great number of studies have proved that the fiber in our diet slightly but conclusively lowers our risk of colon cancer.[54]

All in all, directly or indirectly, it would seem that we might assume that most fruits and vegetables are good for our health.

So does that mean there are no problems with fruits and vegetables? Is there no caveat to all that's been said? Are we quite sure about this conclusion?

NITRATES, PESTICIDES, AND TOXIC SUBSTANCES

As happens every time, we need once more to curb our enthusiasm a little. Fruits and vegetables are, in fact, the main source of carcinogens in our food for most of us. Alongside the metals and PCBs found in some fish, and the arsenic and other delightful stuff in tap or bottled water, we have to acknowledge that it's actually in fruits and vegetables where we find the most carcinogenic compounds, which may be nitrates, nitrites, pesticides, fungicides, or other chemicals. We now know, for example, that 70% of the nitrates in our food comes from vegetables.

Knowing that 5% to 20% of these nitrates will be turned into nitrites by the bacterial flora in our alimentary canal, and that these nitrites then get transformed into highly carcinogenic N-nitroso compounds (NOCs), we can already grasp why we're quite right to be somewhat prudent.[55]

But that's not all. A recent Canadian study showed that there were pesticide residues in 15% of commercially available fruits and vegetables.[56] Even more recently, the Environmental Working Group (EWG) published a study on the pesticides in forty-seven fruits and vegetables, a study based on eighty-seven thousand tests carried out

TABLE 6-10

FRUITS AND VEGETABLES WITH THE MOST
AND THE LEAST PESTICIDES[57]

Dirty Dozen Plus™	Clean Fifteen™
Apples	Avocadoes
Strawberries	Sweet corn
Grapes	Pineapples
Celery	Cabbage
Peaches	Sweet peas—frozen
Spinach	Onions
Sweet bell peppers	Asparagus
Nectarines—imported	Mangoes
Cucumbers	Papaya
Cherry tomatoes	Kiwi
Snap peas—imported	Eggplant
Potatoes	Grapefruit
Hot peppers	Cantaloupe
	Cauliflower
	Sweet potatoes

between 2000 and 2007—with alarming results (see Table 6-10). Someone eating the twelve most-contaminated fruits and vegetables (Dirty Dozen Plus™) would consume on average ten pesticides per day. Whereas eating the fifteen least-contaminated fruits and vegetables (Clean Fifteen™) would expose a person to less than two pesticides per day, on average.[58]

As part of the Pesticide Data Program set up by the U.S. Department of Agriculture in 1991, the department tested 8,172 samples of produce on sale in the United States in 2007. The testing revealed that 97.9% of the samples had pesticide levels higher than the guidelines. This was particularly true for celery, peaches, carrots, and cherries, and the samples included a remarkable number of different, potentially toxic substances.

In its report published in 2013 *Shopper's Guide to Pesticides in Produce*, the EWG provides us with some quite staggering information: "The most recent (2010) round of tests (made by USDA and FDA) show that 68% of food samples had detectable pesticide residue." Similarly, the report points out that:

- 98% of conventional apples have detectable levels of pesticide
- Domestic blueberries tested positive for 42 different pesticide residues
- 78 different pesticides were found on lettuce samples
- Every single nectarine USDA tested had measurable pesticide residues.[59]

TABLE 6-11

PESTICIDE DATA PROGRAM RESULTS FOR FRUITS AND VEGETABLES[60]

	No residues	Percentage of residues detected	Products with excessive levels	The least-contaminated produce
Fruit and vegetables	2.1%	97.9%	All	Bananas Blueberries Broccoli Tomatoes

BASIC ADVICE ON PREPARING
FRUITS AND VEGETABLES

So what should we do?

Apart from choosing organic produce, you must remember to wash your fruits and vegetables thoroughly and for a long time. Do bear in mind that rinsing them will get rid of some but not all of the pesticides, unless you wash them in soapy water. This is because many pesticides are fat soluble but not water soluble.

Your exposure to pesticides will be greatly reduced if you peel your produce, but then you will often lose much of the nutritional goodness, in particular, vitamins and minerals.[61] If you discard the outer leaves of cabbages, lettuce, and salad leaves, you generally do not need to worry about the pesticides. Sometimes brushing your fruits or vegetables can improve the situation, but of course don't try this with raspberries and strawberries.

Chapter 7

....

Fats and Cooking Methods

....

Let's start what you can imagine is a particularly important chapter with this conundrum: Chinese women living in Hong Kong have one of the highest rates of lung cancer anywhere in the world.[1] We also find a dreadfully high incidence elsewhere, in most large Chinese cities and for Chinese women living in Singapore, Malaysia, Hawaii, and Japan. Yet all the epidemiological studies show that only 36% of women with lung cancer in Hong Kong, and barely 24% in Shanghai, smoke.[2] Why is this so? Is there some sort of curse that plagues and decimates these unlucky Chinese women, most of whom have never smoked, and makes them suffer one of the most dreadful of cancers?

Don't rack your brains any further. Although the answer is quite incredible, it has now been completely authenticated: it is because of the way they cook their food. As unlikely as it may seem, this terrible loss of life has nothing to do with cigarettes or even urban pollution— absolutely nothing at all. It is because Chinese women cook with a wok, using potentially carcinogenic oils.

We'll come back to this later in the chapter, so that you get a full explanation about this worrying phenomenon, which I'm sure most of you were quite unaware of.

FATS AND CANCER

Let's start at the beginning.

Do fats help increase or decrease our risk of getting cancer? And if they do increase it, which cancers are we talking about? Does the way we cook our food make it carcinogenic, and does this happen whether we cook with or without fats? The scientific literature on this topic is so prolific, and so many different misleading rumors abound, that to try and answer these three questions is quite a challenge, but let's try to gain a clearer understanding together.

If there is one food family you're probably ill acquainted with, it is the family of fats. When I hear people talking about fats, I get the impression at times that they are talking about some huge stepfamily where everyone and everything is confused.

You are told to eat oils with unsaturated fatty acids because they're healthier.[3] That's your first mistaken notion: you believe these oils are good and contain fewer calories. But that's not the case. All these oils contain almost 100% fat and must be consumed in moderation. To avoid cancer as much as possible, first and foremost you must remember that because of the amount of calories they contain, whether high in unsaturated fatty acids or not, fats are likely to make you put on weight. As we will see later, this is a huge risk factor as far as cancer is concerned.

Next, the second error comes from thinking that anything that is a plant is less harmful and that vegetable oils are therefore healthier than the saturated fats found in meat and dairy products. Well, this too isn't true and is a big mistake. Remember that the worst poisons—tobacco, in particular—are found in the plant kingdom. Many vegetable oils contain just as many saturated fatty acids as animal products.

Does this mean that it is best, as some suggest, to avoid eating fats altogether? Again, this is not a good idea because certain vitamins and trace elements, especially some that prevent cancer, are liposoluble. If you eat no fats, you cannot derive their benefits, which will damage your health. To eat well, lipids or fats should make up around 30% to 35% of your daily energy intake.[4]

TABLE 7-1

COMPARISON OF CONSTITUENTS OF DIFFERENT FATS[5,6]

Fat	Calories (kcal/ 100 g)	Lipids (g/100 g)	Saturated fatty acids (SFAs) (g/100 g)	Monounsat- urated fatty acids (MUFAs) (g/100 g)	Polyunsat- urated fatty acids (PUFAs) (g/100 g)	Cholesterol (mg/100 g)
Butter, salt free	717	81.11	51.368	21.021	3.043	215
Goose fat	900	99.8	27.700	56.700	11.000	100
Margarine	713	80.17	14.224	36.435	26.741	0
Lard	902	100.00	39.200	45.100	11.200	95
Peanut oil	884	100.00	16.900	46.200	32.000	0

Fine. But which lipids should we eat?

There are four types of fatty acids:

1. Polyunsaturated fatty acids (PUFAs), which are found in many vegetable oils (soy, corn, sunflower), oily fish (salmon, mackerel, smelt, herrings, and oysters), fish oils, linseed and sunflower seeds, soy, and some walnuts.
2. Monounsaturated fatty acids (MUFAs), which are found in olive, canola, and high oleic sunflower oil, avocadoes, pears, and some nuts (cashews, pecans, almonds, peanuts, etc.).
3. Saturated fatty acids (SFAs), which are found in coconut, palm, and palm kernel oil, animal fats (pork, beef), butter, and cheese.
4. Trans fatty acids (TFAs), which are found in their natural state in small quantities in some food items (dairy products, beef, and lamb). They also form when canola and soy oils are refined and when liquid oil is processed into semi-solid fats, as with margarine.

Foods made with fats or oils with a high content of saturated fatty acids or trans-fats often have very appealing flavors and textures. Oils

TABLE 7-2

BREAKDOWN FOR DIFFERENT FATTY ACIDS IN VARIOUS OILS[7]

Oil	Calories (kcal/ 100 g)	Lipid content (g/100 g)	SFAs (g/100 g)	MUFAs (g/100 g)	PUFAs (g/100 g)
Peanut	884	100.00	16.900	46.200	32.000
Virgin olive	884	100.00	13.808	72.961	10.523
Rapeseed	884	100.00	7.365	63.276	28.142
Walnut	884	100.00	9.100	22.800	63.300
Grapeseed	884	100.00	9.600	16.100	69.900
Soybean	884	100.00	15.650	22.783	57.740
Sunflower	884	100.00	10.300	19.500	65.700
Retail mixture of oils	884	100.00	14.367	48.033	33.033

high in polyunsaturated and monounsaturated fatty acids are high in omega-3, omega-6, and omega-9.

OMEGA-3 FATTY ACIDS

Now that we've completed our short survey and you know about different oils, you're going to ask me, Which oils should I eat?

I'm sorry, I sense that you're not going to like the answer, but I have to tell you plainly and squarely that there is no proof whatsoever that omega-3 protects us from cancer[8] (or omega-6 or omega-9 for that matter). To put it simply, for humans at least, there is absolutely no proof we can mention here that is sufficiently convincing from a scientific point of view.

Indirect studies looking at the consumption of fish rich in omega-3, for example may have shown an impact on some cancers. However, unfortunately, other studies appearing soon after contradicted these effects.[9] Lastly, in its famous 2007 report, the World Cancer Research Fund only mentions omega-3 once as a component in food that actually protects us from cancer.[10]

In fact, the situation may be even worse, because when exposed to light, omega-3 and omega-6 have an annoying tendency to turn into far less healthy substances. They transform into toxic compounds such as free radicals and lipid peroxides, which particularly attack the genetic material contained in our cells.[11] And this happens simply because oils rich in omega-3 and omega-6 are especially unstable when exposed to light, and they end up going rancid, thereby transforming good unsaturated fatty acids into carcinogenic agents. Although you might often think you are using oil good for your health, once it has come into contact with light, this oil turns rancid and becomes loaded with carcinogenic lipid peroxides. A piece of advice: store these oils away from light, place them in light-resistant containers, and use them up quickly (buy small bottles!).

To get back to omega-3, although several trials on humans are continuing to try to show a preventive effect for certain cancers, to date none of these studies allow us to conclude that this effect has been proved. Moreover, in 2006, in a famous paper published in the renowned *Journal of the American Medical Association*, or *JAMA*, one of the foremost experts on this subject, Professor C. H. MacLean, stated that there was little likelihood of omega-3 consumption reducing the risk of cancer.[12]

WHAT HAPPENS WHEN WE HEAT OILS?

In addition to light, heat if not used properly can also be a factor for toxicity in oils, of whatever type. The principle is simple. The more unstable the oil (for example, oils high in polyunsaturated or monounsaturated fatty acids), the less it can resist high temperatures. With heat, the fatty substances gradually change because of the action of oxygen and air. The oil then colors and becomes viscous, and foam appears. This is the smoke point (see Table 7-3), and it is precisely at this moment that the oil becomes harmful. The glycerol in the fatty substances breaks down into acrolein; there is an acrid smell, and the lipid peroxides that our cells so detest appear in large numbers.[13] The oil then becomes carcinogenic. Numerous substances that promote cancer appear in oils heated to high temperatures; in fact, more than fifty volatile organic compounds have been found, some of which are known for being powerful mutagens (capable of making genetic information in cells mutate) and for being verifiably carcinogenic to humans. They include benzene, benzo[a]pyrene, anthocene, acrolein, and formaldehyde[14] (see Table 3-2).

Even if you aren't an expert, you have to admit that there's nothing remotely reassuring about these names. And you're quite right. They are terrible carcinogens, capable within a few minutes of permanently turning one of your normal cells into a cancerous cell. Once this cell appears, it will usually be too late to stop it, because regardless of what you do, hidden in your body, the cell will start dividing and multiplying. One cell will produce two, and then four, eight, sixteen, thirty

TABLE 7-3

SMOKE POINTS FOR VARIOUS OILS[15]

Oil	Smoke point (°C/°F)
Almond	216/421
Peanut	227/441
Peanut, virgin	160/320
Rapeseed, refined	204/399
Rapeseed, semi-refined	177/351
Rapeseed, virgin	107/351
Macadamia	199/390
Hazelnut	221/430
Walnut, virgin	160/320
Olive, extra virgin	160/320
Palm	240/464
Grape seed	216/421
Sesame, virgin	177/351
Soy, virgin	160/320
Sunflower, virgin oleic	160/320
Sunflower, virgin	107/351

two, sixty-four, and so on and so on, until one day you'll notice that you have a cancer.

This is the reason why the World Health Organization has classified cooking with oil at a high temperature as a group 2A carcinogenic process (that is, probable)[16] (see Table 3-2). It depends, of course, on the oil you use and the cooking temperature. There is also the problem of using the same oil over and over again. Don't think that this is a rare occurrence. In France, the second study published by the Directorate General for Competition, Consumer Affairs and Repression of Fraud (DGCCRF),[17] based on 2,358 checks carried out in all types of restaurants, showed that a sixth of the oils used were deteriorated and dangerous, and that many of them should have been changed long ago. It is quite likely that the situation in the United States is not so very different, though we have not come across an equivalent study published by an American institution.

COOKING UTENSILS

What you simply need to know is that when you place fresh food into a *flat* frying pan with some oil, the food is bound to release some of the water it contains into the oil. This water stops the oil from reaching a dangerous temperature. Another good thing about using this type of utensil is that the heat is distributed evenly across the flat surface of the pan.

However, if you use a wok, as cooks do in many Asian countries, the temperature in the bottom of the wok is likely to exceed 240°C (464°F),[18] causing polycyclic aromatic amines to appear that are highly carcinogenic. Earlier we mentioned a few of the most well-known and toxic amines for humans.

There is lots of evidence to confirm this data, not only from experiments on animals but, as I told you in chapter 1, from studies on humans too. We know, for example, that it is this phenomenon that provides the answer to the conundrum presented at the start of this chapter. We can even measure the risk level for lung cancer in Asian women based on how many meals a week they cook with a wok and how many years they have been using a wok.[19] A recent study of staff working in twenty-three Asian restaurants also showed a greater risk of cancer from cooking-oil fumes for Chinese chefs than for their serving staff.

ARE ALL OILS THE SAME?

Of course, the oil you use also plays a role. First, the smoke point is not the same for all oils, as we can see from Table 7-3. Next, how carcinogenic the oil is depends on the degree of fat saturation. There has been confirmation that there is a problem of carcinogenic polycyclic aromatic hydrocarbons appearing in oils that are heated to a high temperature, in particular with rapeseed, perilla, and hempseed oils.[20]

For example, if we deem cooking in a wok with linseed oil as the least dangerous (although it has been conclusively proved that the wok produces lung cancer even with this oil), and instead use rapeseed oil, that increases the risk of lung cancer by 65%. Were we to use perilla or hempseed oil, the risk would be multiplied by 325%. Peanut oil, by the way, appears to be the least dangerous to use in a wok.[21]

Once again, I am not suggesting that we totally ban woks and rapeseed oil for good. Still, you do need to know this information so that you can choose your oil according to the type of cooking you will be doing. You can then avoid behaviors, such as smoking and cooking with a wok, that considerably increase your risk of lung cancer.

However, there may be solutions for detoxifying the mutagenic and carcinogenic effect of polycyclic aromatic hydrocarbons. Indeed, in 2002, some Taiwanese authors showed that a good dose of quercetin (which we have already looked at, but will discuss again in the chapter on dietary supplements) could inhibit this harmful effect, opening the way for a useful means of preventing it.[22]

Now you are probably anxious, having found out just how carcinogenic fats can be when exposed to light or heated to a high temperature, in addition to them being fattening, and the elevated risk of cancer associated with them.

ACRYLAMIDE, A CARCINOGEN PRODUCED WHEN SOME FOODS ARE COOKED

I am afraid that I am about to make you even more anxious now, because we have to talk about another, extraordinarily carcinogenic substance, acrylamide, which appears when we cook certain foods.

Acrylamide, classified by the World Health Organization as a proven carcinogen for humans[23] (see Table 3-2), is beginning to worry many health organizations, including the French Food Safety Agency (AFSSA)[24]; Health Canada,[25] which has launched a vast sampling plan for an acrylamide-monitoring program; and the European Food Safety Authority.[26]

What exactly is acrylamide? Acrylamide is a chemical compound. When specific foods are being heated to high temperatures, during which the sugars in the foods being cooked combine with certain amino acids present in the foods, a chemical reaction can take place. In this case, the reaction, known as the "Maillard reaction," is likely to produce acrylamide, which is highly carcinogenic if the amino acid that it reacts with is asparagines.[27] Quite logically, if you heat a food in high in asparagines to a high temperature, some carcinogenic acrylamide is likely to appear. Asparagines, for example, makes up 40% of all the amino acids in potato chips, 14% of those in wheat flour, and 18% of those in high-protein, rye-based products.[28]

The U.S. Food and Drug Administration recently presented a report based on its 2006 Total Diet Study, which analyzed data taken from hundreds of samples of common foods produced by the food-processing industry and frequently bought at supermarkets.[29]

For obvious reasons, no brand names are mentioned, but as you can see from the 2006 Total Diet Study results, at times the data can give us quite a fright!

The samples taken from dairy products contain extremely low acrylamide levels, ranging from 0 to 18 mg/kg. By way of comparison, French fries and potato chips could reach up to 393 mg/kg and butter crackers, 336 mg/kg. As for teething biscuits for babies, levels could reach 381 mg/kg. For a substance as carcinogenic as acrylamide, this is quite something!

TABLE 7-4

ACRYLAMIDE LEVELS FOUND IN STORE-BOUGHT
PRODUCTS, BY PRODUCT TYPE[30]

Products	Average acrylamide content (mg/kg)
Coffee, made from grounds	Not detected
Pretzels (hard)	470
Corn tortilla chips	355
Potato chips	346
Potatoes, french-fried, fast food	393
Apple pie, fresh/frozen	18
Chocolate-chip cookies	229
Muffins, fruit or plain	28
Doughnuts, cake type	26
Shredded-wheat cereal	237
Cornflakes, cereal	50
Crackers, saltine	39
Bagels, plain, toasted	32
Candy bars, milk chocolate, plain	17
Peanut butter, creamy	54
Baby food, teething biscuits	381
Infant formula, milk-based, high iron, ready-to-feed	Not detected
Chili con carne/beans, canned	55
Beef and vegetable stew, canned	22
Ice cream, vanilla, light	18
Milk shake, chocolate, fast food	Not detected

We have looked at the risks connected with certain ways of cooking, types of oils, and specific products. What about the effect of eating
fats, in general, and our risk of cancer? And, to round off, what do we
know about other ways of cooking?

Once again, apart from the risk of gaining weight from eating fats,
which are always laden with calories, there is no convincing evidence to
lead us to believe with any certainty that the other fats that have been
studied, and butter especially, might have either a positive or a negative
effect regarding the risk of cancer.

TABLE 7-5

**SELECTED LIST OF PRODUCTS WITH REDUCED
ACRYLAMIDE LEVELS[31]**

Products	Country	Average acrylamide level (µg/kg)
Wheat-based sweet biscuit	France	<10
Dark chocolate	Switzerland	<10
Dairy desserts	France	<10
Madeleine	France	<10
Sponge pudding	France	<10
Fermented dairy products	France	<10
French toast	France	10
Pancakes, frozen, heated	United States	<17
Lasagna	Switzerland	<20
Apple pie	United States	<20
Candy bars, milk chocolate, plain	United States	<20
Burritos, Mexican (take-out)	United States	<20
Muffins	United States	<30
Chocolate patisserie	France	32
Bagels, plain toasted	United States	<40
French fries (pre-fried frozen product)	France	<50
Ice cream, regular, vanilla	United States	Not detected
Coffee, ground	United States	Not detected

Some good news at last!

Unfortunately, the other news is more negative and was mentioned before when we talked about meat and cooking on a barbecue or, more generally, grilling food. What is ironic is that so many people think that to eat healthily, they should always opt for grilled fish or steak.

In fact, this way of cooking is definitely dangerous for your health, as far as cancer is concerned. As we have seen, the process of grilling is linked to the effect of high temperatures on organic (biolog-

TABLE 7-6

SELECTED LIST OF PRODUCTS WITH HIGH ACRYLAMIDE LEVELS[32]

Products	Country	Average acrylamide content (μg/kg)
Cookies	France	550
Instant coffee	Switzerland	567
Honey breakfast cereals	France	410
Chicory	Switzerland	1,300
Crackers	France	250
Low-fat corn chips	France	245
French fries	Switzerland	2,600
Gingerbread	France	300
Fried, potato-based savory product	France	900
Extruded, savory snacks	France	600
Pretzels	United States	470
Crackers, butter type	United States	336
Potato chips	United States	346
Corn tortilla chips	United States	355
Potatoes, French-fried, fast food	United States	393
Shredded-wheat cereal	United States	237
Baby food, teething biscuits	United States	381

ical) products, which produces quantities of neoformed compounds like heterocyclic amines and polycyclic aromatic hydrocarbons, two types of highly carcinogenic products. This happens because the meat or fish comes into contact with flames that reach temperatures above 500°C, or 932°F.

However, according to the American Cancer Society, you don't have to give up your grill to stay healthy. You just need to choose sensible foods and use the right techniques. According to the society's website:[33]

- Choose lean cuts of meat and trim any excess fat. Fat dripping onto hot coals causes smoke that contains potential carcinogens. Less fat means less smoke.
- Line the grill with foil and poke small holes in it so the fat can still drip off, but the amount of smoke coming back onto the meat is lower.
- Avoid charring meat or eating parts that are especially burned and black—they have the highest concentrations of heterocyclic amines.
- Add colorful vegetables and fruit to the grill. Many of the chemicals that are created when meat is grilled are not formed during the grilling of vegetables or fruits, so you can enjoy the grilled flavor worry-free. They're also naturally low in fat and usually need only a short time over heat to gain a terrific smoky flavor. Red, yellow, and green peppers, yellow squash, mushrooms, red onions, and pineapple—all grill well and make healthy additions to your plate.

LET ME SAY THIS AGAIN: I am not suggesting you give up your barbecue for good and throw it away. I simply mean that you need to use it sparingly, a few times a year. In the meantime, you should avoid eating grilled meat too often.

Whenever you can, it is best to try eating your steak as steak tartare, like 28% of the French population does. If you are going to cook your meat, then try cooking it a little less well done; over 60% of French people eat their meat rare. Why not have a go at eating your fish raw too? In France, one person in eight eats fish this way (let me remind you though to avoid red tuna, swordfish, and salmon).[34]

Chapter 8

·················

Sugars and Sugar Products
DON'T CUT THEM OUT ALTOGETHER

··

Quite recently, one of my friends, a well-known humorist, addressed this question to me over dinner: "You agree, don't you, that white sugar refined with that process using dog bones is terribly carcinogenic?" I have to confess that for a moment, I thought he was joking. But I cannot tell you how amazed I was when I realized that all the guests around me agreed with him totally.

Apart from the fact that sugar refining does *not* involve any dog-bone powder, I believe that it is because of such ignorance that we really need to put the record straight about sugar—which means devoting a whole chapter to it.

Ah, sugar! Just say the word "sugar," and I'm sure that a good many of you can already see candies, cakes, cookies, chocolate, and all sorts of treats pass before your eyes, whereas the mention of "steak" or "cauliflower" does not quite get you dreaming to the same extent.

The taste of sugar soothes us, it does us good, it makes us want to take just another tiny mouthful, and then another . . . If we listened to ourselves, and there were no restrictions on the amount of sugar we should eat, confectioners would be working flat-out all year round. These sugary foods evoke nostalgia for our childhood, for those jam

TABLE 8-1

THE SWEETENING POWER OF DIFFERENT SWEETENERS

Sweetener	Relative sweetening power
Acesulfame (E940)	130–200
Aspartame (E951)	200
Fructose	110–120
Glucose	70
Honey	100
Invert sugar	100–110
Lactose	30
Saccharin	300–500
Sucrose (benchmark)	100

and jelly recipes passed down from one generation to the next, for the comfort of mother and family.

Why? Because taste, one of our five senses, is linked to the receptors in our tongue and mouth. Babies have seven thousand of them, but by the age of sixty our average number has dwindled to two thousand. Each one of these receptors is specific to a basic taste: salty, sweet, sour, or bitter. The sweet receptors are not only more numerous, but also the first ones to appear in the fetus as it forms in its mother's womb.[1]

EATING SUGAR AND THE RISK OF CANCER

Now, is there any connection between eating sugars or sweeteners and the risk of cancer?[2]

One way of hinting at the answer to this question is to point out that the World Cancer Research Fund's famous global report on food and cancer, to which we have repeatedly made reference in this book, and which is over six hundred pages, devotes only one page to sugars and sweeteners.[3] Barely one page . . .

I believe it is the case that people like you, who have gone out and bought an anticancer diet book, want to know more. You want to form your own opinion based on the relevant information and evidence you have read, understood, and digested, and after you have then applied common sense to scrutinize the whole corpus of information. Ultimately you will draw your own conclusions and adopt new eating habits that will better control your risk of cancer as well as any risk for those who are dear to you, especially your children.

Let's start then by looking at real sugar products.

What do we know, and how have we managed to get to a point where pseudo-specialists can claim that sugar is carcinogenic, even though the most respected body in the world in its lengthy report has reached the very opposite conclusion? Quite simply what these pseudo-specialists are doing is fear mongering. They are mixing up ideas in a way that is scientifically unacceptable.

The effects of insulin and IGF1

What do we actually know about sugar? The one thing we know is that being overweight or obese increases the risk of cancer. Nowadays, this fact is beyond dispute, and very soon you will reach the full chapter we devote to it.

But based on this scientifically correct information, why have some people forbidden you to eat sugar? It is somewhat complicated, but I'm going to try to explain it to you. There is a very important hormone in our bodies that controls what happens to the sugar and fat we eat. This hormone is insulin, and it decides what our bodies absorb and what is involved in our energy metabolism. Insulin makes us either store sugar when it is relatively overabundant (as when we have a rich diet, or little energy is being burnt up), or, if the situation is reversed, use the sugar that has been stored, primarily in the liver and muscles. Insulin also helps create a second energy store in our fat, and should the need arise—for example, in times of famine or if we are following a weight-loss diet—insulin will take whatever it needs from this fat to make more sugar.

You can see that this hormone is essential. However, if a person is obese, insulin is unable to do its job properly. It is almost as if the insulin becomes overwhelmed while attempting to control all the energy we are absorbing from a too rich diet, while at the same time controlling the fat we store away, basically everywhere in our bodies. So just like anything else, if insulin gets overloaded with work, it can no longer cope. Then what happens?

TABLE 8-2

AMOUNT OF CARBOHYDRATES AND LIPIDS IN VARIOUS SUGAR PRODUCTS[4]

Products	Per 100 g of product			
	Calories (kcal)	Total carbohydrates (g)	Sugars (g)	Lipids (g)
Butter cookies	467	69.80	20.24	18.80
Hard candies	394	98.00	62.90	0.20
Brownies	405	63.9	36.61	16.3
Cheesecake	321	25.5	21.8	22.5
Milk chocolate	535	57.5	51.50	29.40
Dark chocolate (70–85% cocoa)	598	45.90	23.99	42.63
Jams and preserves (average)	278	68.86	48.50	0.07
Chocolate-chip cookies	474	63.86	35.14	23.31
Vanilla ice cream	207	23.60	21.22	11.00
Iced chocolate doughnuts	417	57.40	31.92	19.90
Cream puffs, éclairs	334	37.43	22.05	18.52
Fructose[5]	380	95	95	0
Fruitcake	324	61.60	27.42	9.10
Peanut butter	520	35.65	9.28	34
Vanilla wafers	441	73.60	37.50	15.2
Honey	304	82.40	82.12	0
Carrot cake	292	43.7	21.1	11.3
Chocolate-hazelnut spread	541	62.16	54.05	29.73
Sugar	387	99.98	99.98	0
Dutch apple pie	290	44.54	22.02	11.50

Our pancreas starts secreting more and more insulin in increasing amounts as it tries to cope. Then there will be lots of insulin in the blood, a condition we call "hyperinsulinemia." At a certain point, and this is what we observe in people who are too fat, there can be an overload, resulting in what is called "type 2 diabetes" (different from type 1 diabetes, where the pancreas stops producing insulin).

If insulin is present in such great quantities, other than simply managing your sugar, it starts to take on other roles, either with the sugar circulating in your blood (glycemia) or with the sugar stored. Insulin becomes a factor stimulating cell growth or cell proliferation.[6] It does this for all cells, normal or cancerous.

When there is too much insulin, it will also get the liver to secrete another substance, one that stimulates cell proliferation: IGF1 (insulin-like growth factor). In certain circumstances, insulin will even imitate IGF1 and take its place, stimulating cell multiplication to an even greater degree.

However, the effect of IGF1, or insulin when it imitates IGF1 and takes its place, potentially can be very dangerous as far as the risk of cancer is concerned, because when it is influenced by carcinogenic toxins, this substance encourages normal cells to turn into cancerous cells. It also inhibits the suicide of cancerous cells (apoptosis), and, lastly, it directly stimulates the cells' capacity to divide and multiply.[7]

In a more indirect but equally dangerous way, IGF1 and excess insulin boost the production of sexual hormones,[8] such as estrogens, also risking to stimulate growth in potentially cancerous cells hidden in a breast. The same is true for male hormones and the risk of prostate cancer. What we have here is a mechanism, thoroughly identified and understood, that explains the link between obesity and the risk of cancer, as we'll see in a later chapter.

But, you'll ask me, what about sugar? Well, sugar, in this case, has absolutely nothing to do with it, at least when we eat it as a food. As I told you earlier, ideas get spuriously mixed up. Sugar as a food is not involved in this in any way whatsoever. The mix-up comes from the connection we all make in our minds between insulin, diabetes, and sugar.

Let's go further. As you can well imagine, numerous studies have been carried out to discover whether there is not in fact some small connection between sugar itself and certain cancers. Studies dealing with six cancers—prostate, colon, ovarian, breast, pancreatic, and uterine—have indeed been undertaken. To simplify things, let's make it clear straightaway that no serious study has been able to obtain any reproducible results for a connection between eating sugar and pancreatic,[9] prostate,[10] ovarian or uterine[11] cancer.

For breast cancer, two major cohort studies have had negative results. The first involved almost sixty thousand Swedish women monitored for more than fifteen years. It showed that the 2,952 women who ended up getting breast cancer while the cohort was being monitored did not eat any more sugar than the 57,000 women in the cohort who did not develop breast cancer.[12] The second study included just over sixty thousand women, who were monitored over ten years but who were already menopausal. This study showed that being overweight or having an expanded waistline (an indirect way of checking for weight problems) correlated with the risk of breast cancer,[13] but there was no connection between the amount of sugar eaten and breast cancer.

Lastly, a vast study that averaged out all the studies published in this area up to 2008 reached a final conclusion that there was no significant link between the amount of sugar consumed and the risk of getting breast cancer, either before or after menopause.[14]

There remains colon cancer. If we look at the conclusions from two large prospective cohort studies,[15] involving over 130,000 people who were monitored for almost twenty years, we see that for women there is no link between eating sugar and colorectal cancer. There might be a slightly higher risk for men but only for overweight men and only if they consume sugar in great quantities and only if that sugar is in the form of fructose and sucrose.

Honestly, given what we already know about the risks of being overweight, it is difficult to apportion all the blame to sugar for people who already have an elevated risk of cancer.

Finally, all the studies published on this subject were recently reviewed, and the findings make it possible once and for all to discount any link between the amount of sugars consumed and an increased risk of colorectal cancer.[16]

Better still, the huge Multiethnic Cohort Study, which involved over 191,000 adults, recently arrived at the opposite conclusion. For women at any rate, eating lots of carbohydrates seems to protect them from colorectal cancer[17]—on the condition that they stay slim, of course!

WHAT ABOUT SWEETENERS?

To round off this chapter, let's discuss what we should do about the sweeteners that everyone calls "artificial sugars."

Aspartame

In 1996, a rumor about aspartame being toxic spread across the Internet; it was alleged that this sweetener was carcinogenic.

Where are we at now, more than fifteen years later? First, aspartame is not an artificial product. Discovered in 1965, it is in fact the combination of two amino acids: L-aspartic acid and L-phenylalanine acid. It provides no energy (zero calories); on the other hand, it is two hundred times sweeter than sugar and an excellent palliative for eating sugar. Since 1981, more than sixteen years after it was discovered, the World Health Organization and the Food and Agriculture Organization certified aspartame, without any restriction, as totally harmless to human health. Both institutions recommend that consumption should not exceed 40 mg/kg/day (today, the U.S. Food and Drug Administration has even increased this level to 50 mg/kg/day). For a man weighing 175 pounds, this means a daily intake of 3,200 mg—that is, over 150 packets of sweeteners! Just for comparison, a diabetic using only sweeteners all day long still would not take more than 10 mg/kg/day.[18] There really is no cause for concern.

Moreover, the American Cancer Society's *Guidelines on Nutrition and Physical Activity for Cancer Prevention* put it clearly:

Do non-nutritive sweeteners or sugar substitutes cause cancer? There is no proof that these sweeteners, at the levels consumed in human diets, cause cancer. Aspartame, saccharin, and sucralose are a few of the non-nutritive sweeteners approved for use by the FDA. Current evidence does not show a link between these compounds and increased cancer risk. Some animal studies have suggested that their use may be linked with an increased risk of cancers of the bladder and brain, or of leukemias and lymphomas, but studies in humans show no increased cancer risk. People with the genetic disorder phenylketonuria, however, should avoid aspartame in their diets.[19]

Agave syrup and stevia

Lastly, what about certain other sweeteners we might use, such as agave syrup and stevia? As for agave syrup, extracted from Mexican cacti that, as it happens, are also used to produce tequila, it has been said that it is better than sugar. What nonsense! First, since everything actually concurs to prove that sugar is healthy, why substitute one healthy product with another? Next, when we take into account the antioxidant properties of a whole range of sweeteners, we realize that agave syrup is on a par with sugar,[20] and far worse than maple syrup or honey. Finally, when I asked my friend Professor Jaime de la Garza, chairman of the Mexican National Cancer Institute, if, by any chance Mexican Indians, who according to age-old tradition use agave syrup to sweeten their foods, had less cancers than other ethnic groups in Mexico, he laughed in my face and confirmed that this was not so.

What should we think of stevia, which has recently come on the scene? Stevia has sweetening power 140 to 250 times greater than that of saccharin, depending on the type of plant used.[21] As far as stevia studies are concerned, I have not yet had enough time to assess them, so I prefer to exercise caution for the time being and will wait to give my opinion.

Chapter 9
....

What Should We Drink?
....

To keep our bodies alive, it is even more important to be hydrated than to eat. If we don't drink, our chances of survival are far worse than if we were to eat nothing. From the third day without drinking, the symptoms of dehydration start to appear, and if the situation is not quickly remedied, death follows a few days later.

Why? Because our bodies are 65% water,[1] in children the percentage is even higher.

In developed countries, we are very lucky to have no problem accessing relatively safe drinking water. However, we should remember that for over 20% of the world's population, finding good drinking water is a problem.[2] According to the World Health Organization, unsafe water kills almost 1.6 million people every year.[3]

IS OUR DRINKING WATER HEALTHFUL?
THE SITUATION IN THE UNITED STATES

In the United States we're told repeatedly that the drinking water is good, whether it comes from the tap or from a bottle, whether spring or mineral water. Is this really true?

According to a report published in 2011 by the U.S. Environ-

TABLE 9-1

**U.S. DRINKING WATER CONTAMINANT AND TECHNICAL
TREATMENT VIOLATIONS IN 2010[4]**

Violation	Number of violations	Water distribution unit		Population supplied	
		Number	Percentage	Number	Percentage
Health-based rules*	19,914	4,862	3.20%	18,997,543	60%
Microbial rules†	13,018	8,512	5.60%	20,343,530	6.4%
Organics rules‡	82	49	0.03%	578,559	0.2%
Inorganics rules‡	5,012	2,750	1.80%	5,185,500	1.6%

* Health-based rules—levels exceeded as regards rules for contaminants and for technical treatments.
† Microbial, health-based rules, applying to all water systems.
‡ Health-based rules in the community water systems (CWS) and the non-transient non-community water systems (NTNCWS).

mental Protection Agency (EPA), there were 152,979 public water distribution systems in 2010, including 51,460 community water systems supplying almost 300 million Americans. According to this same report, health-based violations were recorded for 3% of all the systems, which accounted for water supplied to almost 19 million Americans.[5]

As far as pesticides are concerned, the areas worst affected in France are the Seine and Marne, and Eure and Loire regions. In the United States, some Midwestern states (Kansas, Missouri, and South Dakota) record overall violations that may affect up to one-fourth of the population.[6]

This seems worrying to me, not only because some components in the water (especially the pesticides) are potentially carcinogenic, but also because the water intake for these water distribution units gets inspected in France only once every five years, even for the smallest units, and in the United States, once every three to five years.[7]

Let's consider arsenic, which is classified as a carcinogenic substance by the World Health Organization.

Many studies have provided definitive proof that the arsenic found in water is likely to increase the risk of lung cancer threefold or more—that is, at least a 300% increase in risk. Arsenic might also increase our

TABLE 9-2

ESTIMATED EXPOSURE TO ARSENIC IN DIFFERENT COUNTRIES[8]

Country	Estimated average daily intake
France	Adults: 62 µg/day (up to 163 µg/day)
	Children: 43 µg/day (up to 103 µg/day)
Canada, Poland, United States, United Kingdom	Adults: 17 to 129 µg/day
	Children: 1.3 to 16.0 µg/day

chances of getting bladder cancer and possibly skin cancer too. However, with lung cancer, the evidence is conclusive.[9]

Why not drink bottled mineral water instead? Well, because the statistics on mineral water are no more reassuring. In fact, according to a 1998 survey (the latest one available) from the French National Network for Public Health, arsenic levels exceeded the drinking water standard of 10 µg/L in twenty mineral waters tested—and were even above 50 µg/L in some waters!

In the United States, according to the latest available survey from the Natural Resources Defense Council (NDRC) from 1999, the arsenic level in eight different bottled waters purchased in California exceeded the drinking water standard of 5 µg/L as laid down by California regulations.[10]

Has the situation improved in the meantime? We cannot be sure. We might tell ourselves that water-filter pitchers, so popular nowadays, will solve our problem. But whether dealing with heavy metals, nitrates, pesticides, or organic constituents, these filters are unfortunately far from being a panacea, as Table 9-3 shows.

Nitrates and nitrites

Nitrates are another source of carcinogens that we need to consider. Table 9-4, drawn up from the data published in 2009 by the Environ-

TABLE 9-3

**COMPARING NATURAL MINERAL WATER WITH TAP WATER
FILTERED USING A HOUSEHOLD WATER FILTER**[11]

Parameter	Effects of a water-filter jug	Natural mineral water
Mineral composition	Unknown or modified, variable from one place to another depending on filter-cartridge saturation	Stable and shown on label
Nitrate level	No elimination	< 10 mg/L, stable, shown on label
pH	Modified and variable	Stable, shown on label
Chlorine level	Variable, partially eliminated, 50% effective	Not used, not detectable
Taste, smell	Variable depending on the saturation	Stable, identifiable
Pesticide level	Variable, partially eliminated, 65% effective	In theory, not present
Particles	Released by the filter cartridge	Stable, 30 times less
Pathogens	If contaminated, risk of proliferation	Pathogens absent
Silver	Released by the filter cartridge	Not detectable
Trace minerals	Eliminated, variable	Stable
Organic constituents	Variable, hardly eliminated	Natural, stable, low: < 0.5 mg/L
Heavy metals	Partially eliminated	Lead, mercury, copper, zinc not detectable

mental Working Group, speaks volumes.[12] From time to time, check online for results published by the EPA on the water quality for your town or city.

A note: The data available in the Environmental Working Group trihalomethanes study concerns (THMs) haloacetic acids, (HAAs), nitrates, and arsenic. THMs are four chemicals that are formed along with other disinfection by-products when chlorine or other disinfectants used to control microbial contaminants in drinking water

TABLE 9-4

WATER QUALITY IN SOME MAJOR U.S. CITIES[13]

City	Total trihalomethanes (THMs) (ppb)	Nitrate (ppm)
Phoenix, AZ	38.5	1.7
Los Angeles, CA	34.4	1.5
Los Angeles suburbs, CA	30.8	0.2
San Diego, CA	4.0	0.5
San Francisco, CA	8.6	4.2
San Jose, CA	1.8	4.7
Jacksonville, FL	48.0	0.1
Chicago, IL	16.1	0.3
Indianapolis, IN	33.6	1.2
Boston, MA	3.7	0.1
Las Vegas, NV	62.0	0.9
New York, NY	37.3	0.2
Philadelphia, PA	44.6	2.7
Austin, TX	30.6	0.3
Dallas, TX	32.1	0.3
Houston, TX	20.1	0.2
San Antonio, TX	15.4	1.7

react with naturally occurring organic and inorganic matter in water. The THMs are chloroform, bromodichloromethane, dibromochloromethane, and bromoform.

Cities with the best water

The Environmental Working Group rated big-city (population over 250,000) water utilities based on three factors: the total number of chemicals detected since 2004; the percentage of chemicals found of

those tested; and the highest average level for an individual pollut-
ant, relative to legal limits or national average amounts, including
for the most common pollutants (disinfection by-products, nitrate,
and arsenic).

Since the group's tap-water database was published in December
2009, we have received new test results from several water utilities.

If your water is good, there is no need to spend money on filters
or bottled water. However, if you know that your tap water is contaminated, try to find out which spring or mineral waters are healthy for
you and your family.

TABLE 9-5

**ENVIRONMENTAL WORKING GROUP'S TOP-RATED
AND LOWEST-RATED WATER UTILITIES, 2009[14]**

TOP-RATED WATER UTILITIES	LOWEST-RATED WATER UTILITIES
1. Arlington, TX: Arlington Water Utilities	100. Pensacola, FL: Emerald Coast Water Utility
2. Providence, RI: Providence Water	99. Riverside, CA: City of Riverside Public Utilities
3. Fort Worth, TX: Fort Worth Water Department	98. Las Vegas, NV: Las Vegas Valley Water District
4. Charleston, SC: Charleston Water System	97. Riverside County, CA: Eastern Municipal Water District
5. Boston, MA: Massachusetts Water Resources Authority	96. Reno, NV: Truckee Meadows Water Authority
6. Honolulu, HI: Board of Water Supply (Honolulu/Windward/Pearl Harbor)	95. Houston, TX: City of Houston Public Works
7. Austin, TX: Austin Water Utility	94. Omaha, NE: Metropolitan Utilities District
8. Fairfax County, VA: Fairfax Water	93. North Las Vegas, NV: City of North Las Vegas Utilities Department
9. St. Louis, MO: City of St. Louis Water Division	92. San Diego, CA: San Diego Water Department
10. Minneapolis, MN: City of Minneapolis Water Department	91. Jacksonville, FL: JEA

WHAT ABOUT WINE? IS IT GOOD FOR US OR NOT?

Is wine a risk factor for cancer?

As with water and its high arsenic levels, it is not drinking wine as such that can be dangerous but rather it is drinking *too much* wine.

Trace amounts of arsenic are naturally present in water and have nothing to do with modern-day pollution. If we were to get cancer from simply drinking a little water every day, we would all be long dead.

It's the same with wine. If wine were carcinogenic from the very first glass, as the French National Cancer Institute announced in 2010, we would all have developed cancers of the mouth, liver, colon, and so on, and so would have our ancestors.

So what does science have to say about the link between wine and cancer? We can go back to the literature on the subject and to what the World Cancer Research Fund thinks, as stated in its report in 2007.[15]

Let's start with ear, nose, and throat (ENT) cancer, which I'll simply refer to as "mouth" cancer. The 2007 World Cancer Research Fund report listed twenty-six case-control studies, of which twenty-one are usable. Sixteen of these studies indicated that there is an increase in the risk of mouth cancer for those who are moderate (fewer than two glasses per day for women and fewer than three glasses per day for men) or excessive drinkers. However, the other five studies, which compared the same two groups of individuals, showed that excessive wine consumption reduces the risk of mouth cancer.

By putting all these studies together, we get an average that says that if we drink too much wine, our risk of mouth cancer increases by 2%. Based on the levels of approximation characteristic of case-control studies like those we looked at in our first chapter, we can rest assured that 2% is very low.[16]

Even so, this 2007 report was based on an expert consensus from 2006. It was therefore based on studies that ran up to late 2005 but no further. In June 2006, a momentous discovery was published in the United States, and it has since been confirmed by many other conclusive studies. The discovery that most mouth cancers are in fact caused by a virus, the human papillomavirus (HPV), the same virus that causes cervical cancer and can be transmitted through oral sex.[17] Fortunately, as with cancer of the penis, cervix, and anus, all caused by the same virus, most of us manage to get rid of this virus and develop a local immunity that protects us during future sexual relations. However, some of us are unable to get rid of it. As other risk factors are added over time (smoking, for example), these people could develop mouth cancer.

Incidentally, since anti-HPV vaccinations are now available, there are high hopes that this cancer will be eradicated, along with the three others directly connected with the virus. But let's get back to the studies on wine and mouth cancers. The discovery that over half of mouth cancers could be caused by HPV—something that the scientists did not take into account when setting up their case and control groups—renders the earlier studies unusable.

Instead of examining the evidence for each cancer in excruciating detail, I'm going to simply summarize the rest of the studies about cancer and wine.

For esophageal cancer there are ten case-control studies. Nine of them show a risk, but half of these studies "simply forgot" to take into account whether the individuals in the studies smoked or not, making these studies unusable.[18] As we know, the main risk factor by far for this cancer is smoking tobacco. In any case, the authors of this American report again reached the conclusion that if there were any risk, it would be, on average, scarcely 4%.

With regard to breast, liver, and colon cancer, the evidence is similar.[19] For each one, the risk is 3% to 6% higher for those who drink excessively when compared to moderate drinkers. To my mind, this difference is too slight to be really significant.

RESVERATROL AND ITS PROPERTIES

In fact, when drunk in moderation, wine is extremely good for our health, even as far as cancer is concerned. There is one very simple

TABLE 9-6

RESVERATROL LEVELS (USING HPLC), IN 1997 VINTAGE[20]

Grape variety	Trans-resveratrol (mg/L)	Cis-resveratrol (mg/L)	Total resveratrol (mg/L)
Gamay	40	3	43
Pinot noir	19	6	25
Regent	10	4	14
Gamay rosé	9	3	11
Chardonnay	0.8	1	2

Note: HPLC, high-performance liquid chromatography.

reason for this: wine contains resveratrol,[21] a substance with extraordinary anticancer properties. In fact, red wine, just like grape juice, contains on average 2,000 mg/L of polyphenols (flavonoids, flavins, anthocyanins, and stilbenes such as resveratrol), five to ten times more than what white wine has (which still contains them, so don't worry).[22]

Since resveratrol was discovered in the early 1990s by a team of Japanese scientists, hundreds of studies have been carried out on this antioxidant. Part of the stilbenes family, resveratrol is the vine's response to all the aggression it suffers from pathogens when it is exposed to ultraviolet radiation and ozone. It was resveratrol's anti-inflammatory properties that first came to light. Then resveratrol became recognized as largely responsible for what Serge Renaud, a famous French researcher, named the "French paradox,"[23] or "how to eat fat, drink red wine and not be the leading contenders for cardio-vascular diseases."

More recent studies have focused on resveratrol's anticancer action, as it seems able to act during all stages of cancer: during the initiation stage, when a healthy cell transforms into a cancerous cell; during the promotion stage, when it proliferates at the expense of other healthy cells; and even during the progression stage, when cancerous cells grow.[24]

At each of these three stages the clinical onset of cancer is possible, but resveratrol is capable of inducing a mechanism that can inhibit and block this risk by driving the abnormal cells to suicide (apoptosis), by stimulating the "guardian of the genome" (the p53 protein). It also improves the ability of genes to repair themselves from damage caused by chemical products, carcinogenic radiation, and polycyclic hydrocarbons.[25]

Many experimental models for skin,[26] prostate,[27] colon,[28] pancreatic,[29] and esophageal[30] cancers have provided proof of these properties. This is the reason why many trials are currently being carried out on people to determine the best conditions for resveratrol so that its anticancer properties can be put to the most effective use in preventing the risk of cancer in humans. (The type of alcohol in intoxicating drinks is ethanol. You shouldn't consume more than 30 g—approximately an ounce—per day.)

Is wine bad for our health? Not at all. Quite the opposite, it is probably very good, but nonetheless it should be consumed in moderation.

We have now examined what we need to know about the links between cancer and water and wine. What other drinks do we need to consider?

TABLE 9-7[31]

ETHANOL BY TYPE OF ALCOHOLIC BEVERAGE

Alcoholic Beverage	30 g of ethanol is equivalent to
Champagne	2.5 glasses
Pastis	2 glasses
Rum	5 × 20-mL (.7-oz.) glasses
Wine	2 × 15-cL (5-oz.) glasses
Whisky	Less than 1 × 15-cL (5-oz.) glass

Note: cL, centiliter.

POMEGRANATE JUICE IS A MARVELOUS DRINK

We discussed fruit juices in the chapter on fruits and vegetables, but there are a few more significant points to consider. First of all, fruit juices usually contain a fair amount of calories. We should remember this as we try to avoid becoming overweight, which we now know is a risk factor for many cancers.

For example, we can see from Table 9-8 that grape juice is especially high in calories compared with pineapple juice. When selecting fruit juices, we should bear these hidden calories in mind.

Are all fruit juices good for preventing cancer? Not necessarily.

One popular juice in particular has been associated with an enormous rise in the incidence of malignant melanomas. This skin cancer, which starts out looking like a mole, is probably one of the most terrible. When scarcely four millimeters (over one-eighth of an inch) thick

TABLE 9-8

CALORIES AND CARBOHYDRATES CONTAINED IN DIFFERENT FRUIT JUICES[32]

Type of juice	Calories (kcal/100 mL)	Carbohydrates (g/100 mL)
Pure grape juice	68	15
Mango juice	63	15
Pomegranate juice	61	12
Apricot juice	59	13
Multi-fruit juice	50	12
Pineapple juice	49	12
Pure multi-fruit juice	48	11
Pure orange juice	48	10
Pure apple juice	44	11
Squeezed orange juice	41	9
Pure grapefruit juice	37	8
Soda	44	11

(which for any other cancer is incredibly small), these malignant melanomas will result in death in up to 50% of cases.[33]

Unfortunately, as all the studies have shown, the incidence—that is, the number of new cases diagnosed each year—continues to rise all the time. In developed countries, it is actually doubling every ten years. In the United States, for example, in 1935 there was one case of melanoma per 1,500 inhabitants, and in 2000 there was one case for every 75.[34] And the trend continues upward.

For years researchers the world over have been trying to work out what lies behind this crazy upsurge. For a long time it was thought that the increase was happening because children were being exposed to the sun far too much. It is true that children should not spend too much time unprotected from direct sunlight, especially when they are very young and, in particular, not between eleven in the morning and four in the afternoon. However, even if this cause were indisputable, it could not be the only one. Why? Although there has been an impact on our health because we do seek out the sun, with shorter vacations making us rush out onto the beach, and more air travel allowing ever greater numbers of people to get to a sunny climate, all these sociological changes got under way in the early 1980s. It does not explain why now, thirty years later, there still continues to be such a huge upward trend in the incidence of melanomas.

In 2008, dermatology researchers at the University of Tennessee in Memphis published an extremely interesting study which very seriously suggested that orange juice plays a role in this epidemic.[35] Orange juice does, in fact, contain lots of different furocoumarins and psoralens, which are highly carcinogenic substances for the skin when it is exposed to sunlight. About fifteen or so years ago, this led to a ban on sunscreen products with high levels of bergamot, which contains psoralens.

According to these researchers, perfect parallels have been recorded between the upsurge in the incidence of melanoma and an increased consumption of citrus juices. Furthermore, a recent study carried out on a huge cohort of nurses showed that just drinking lots of orange juice could be statistically linked to the risk of developing a melanoma.[36]

Does this mean that we should stop drinking orange juice?

I don't believe so, but I do think that people predisposed to developing melanoma—that is, blonds or redheads with blue or green eyes, people whose skin burns rather than tans, and people with lots of moles or who are directly related to someone who has had a melanoma—ought not to drink orange juice until we are shown proof to the contrary.

Instead, these people—and most of us—ought to try another fruit juice, and pomegranate juice, which is extremely good for cancer prevention, is an excellent choice. Lots of studies have shown that drinking large quantities of pomegranate juice could slow down the spread of cancerous cells in the prostate, and boost the cell-death phenomenon by blocking the system for cell growth factors and their receptors, especially for one particular growth factor, insulin growth factor, or IGF1.[37, 38]

Similarly, pomegranate fruit extracts have beneficial effects on breast cancers sensitive to female hormones (generally those that are diagnosed after the age of fifty) by inhibiting a key enzyme, aromatase, responsible for producing the estrogens that are potentially capable of stimulating the spread of cancerous cells in breast.[39, 40]

Pomegranates are extremely high in antioxidants, found mainly in their juice and skin.[41] What's more, some research has estimated that pomegranates have an antioxidant action three to four times greater than that of red wine or green tea.[42] These antioxidants also work synergistically; pomegranate juice has greater antioxidant activity than pomegranate tannin extract on its own, or than punicalagin and ellagic acid, two substances found in pomegranates that promote detoxification, on their own.[43]

In addition, of all the juices and drinks tested, pomegranate juice has the greatest anti-proliferation activity on colon-cancer cell lines cultivated in vitro, with an inhibition rate ranging from 30% to 100%.[44] After eight months of administering pomegranate juice orally to mice, in which lung cancer had been induced using chemical carcinogens, the size of their tumors decreased by 66% compared with the tumors in the control group, which got no pomegranate juice.[45]

As we can see, this fruit juice is remarkable, and it is one of the most powerful dietary agents for cancer prevention. It is so powerful, and the experimental data so promising, that studies have already been carried out on humans, with spectacular results.

One of them deserves a mention here. It deals with men with prostate cancer who have already been operated on but who then experienced a recurrence.[46] We know they had a recurrence because a substance in the blood called "prostate-specific antigen" or PSA, increases when prostate cancer recurs. At first, these men whose PSA levels had started to rise were monitored to calculate the speed at which their cancer was spreading again. Then they started drinking pomegranate juice daily, and the rate at which their cancer was spreading slowed down enormously. This deserves to be mentioned because few studies carried out on humans actually suffering from serious cancer have been able to show conclusive, effective results.

Eating pomegranates raw or in salads is good, but the best effects are, in fact, from the juice, and chiefly from the industrially manufactured juices we buy in stores. The industrial process that produces pomegranate juice extracts the water-soluble tannins found in the skin, which might explain why store-bought juices have greater antioxidant activity.[47]

WHAT ARE THE BENEFITS OF HOT DRINKS?

Let's take a look at hot beverages, specifically tea and coffee.

Coffee first. We all remember the study published in 1981, very widely commented on at the time, that seemed to show that drinking coffee regularly could increase the risk of pancreatic cancer[48]—a cancer that we are especially frightened of getting. It turns out there is no need to worry. Dozens of other studies have since invalidated the results: there is no link between coffee and pancreatic cancer. The World Cancer Research Fund report confirmed this.[49]

Even the opposite could be true. If we examine the thirty or so studies about the connection between coffee and colon cancer or the twenty-odd ones on the link between coffee and liver cancer, we get the distinct impression that coffee might well have a preventive effect.[50, 51]

The same goes for breast cancer, at least in premenopausal women. One study showed a significant drop in risk for young women who drink at least four cups a day.[52] Likewise, another study, published in 2006 in the *International Journal of Cancer*, focused on 1,690 women who had inherited a mutated gene that promotes the onset of breast cancer (BRCA genes), and showed that high coffee consumption (six cups per day) considerably lessened their risk of getting this cancer during their lifetime.[53]

We should note that all these effects have only been observed with caffeinated coffee. They have not been recorded for decaffeinated coffee, which seems to be neither good nor bad for us.

WHAT ABOUT TEA?

Tea is one of the most widely drunk beverages in the world, and it is particularly rich in antioxidants. There are, of course, various types of tea, but the one that seems to offer the best protection against cancer is green tea. It has several antioxidants substances, the most important being epigallocatechin-3-gallate (EGCG), which is a powerful polyphenol that inhibits tumor growth by driving cancerous cells to suicide (apoptosis). It also inhibits the formation of new blood vessels that would supply the cancerous cells. The cells are intent on proliferating and are desperate for fresh blood and energy (sugars and oxygen), vital for producing new cells. By preventing the blood vessels from forming around the tumor, EGCG inhibits de facto the risk of cancerous cells using one of these vessels to trigger metastasis.[54]

Some studies have been carried out on humans, notably at the Mayo Clinic in Minnesota. Here the significant clinical benefit of getting patients with certain leukemias or cancers of the lymph nodes (lymphomas) to drink large quantities of green tea was conclusively proved. Another study took place in Atlanta to see if the polyphenols in green tea could boost the effectiveness of some drugs used to treat lung cancers.

Similarly in 2009, a study showed that by regularly drinking large quantities of green tea for at least three months, patients with precancerous mouth lesions could lower their risk of getting actual cancer of the oral cavity by over 50%.[55]

Are all teas healthy? No, one has been proved conclusively to be unhealthy, as it increases the risk of cancer of the esophagus and perhaps of the mouth too. This tea is mate, an infusion of a South American herb, "yerba mate," whose green leaves are toasted and crushed to make a green powder. In Argentina, Paraguay, and Chile this drink is used as a stimulant. It is consumed very hot, all day long, from a small gourd or through a straw. This said, the evidence suggests that there is not a specific carcinogenic substance in mate tea that makes it dangerous, but rather the way in which it is drunk: by a straw, very hot, and throughout the day.[56] Be that as it may, drinking mate tea increases the risk of cancer of the esophagus by around 15%, so it should be avoided.

Chapter 10

....

Dietary Supplements and Nutrients

BENEFICIAL OR HARMFUL?

....

I t's time to take a look at dietary supplements.

Specialist shops, magazines, and books are capitalizing on our infatuation with these substances. We read and hear anything and everything about these products, the packagings of which often promise us miracles: they will make us beautiful, fit, and healthy, stop us from aging, and so on. Yet despite all the impossibilities, we still believe them.

In the United States there are about 56,600 different dietary supplements. Over 50% of American adults used dietary supplements between 2003 and 2006,[1, 2] and more than 30% of children took them regularly between 1999 and 2002.[3]

BOMBARDED WITH SO MANY PRODUCTS and so much information, how do we make sense of it all? How can we be sure that we are doing something good for our health and that we are not using products that are actually more toxic than healthful?

I'm going to help you choose dietary supplements that may be able to help you fight a cancer you already have (or have had) or, even better, stop you from getting one. My role as a cancer specialist is to guide you through the plethora of products on offer, so that you learn to identify which ones are useful and will not harm your health.

I'll start by saying that if there is one thing I would really like you to take away from this chapter, it is that dietary supplements are not drugs, even if they can help you cope better with certain diseases such as cancer.

Dietary supplements cannot cure you. However you combine the products and in whatever doses, a cure from them is quite impossible. From now on, please do not believe anyone who tries to sell you dreams of this sort.

A dietary supplement is meant to improve individuals' well-being and keep them in good health. It may possibly prevent cancer, but it cannot claim to cure any disease, especially a disease as complex and as serious as cancer. Please get rid of any dietary supplement that claims it will cure you of cancer. However, as we will see, dietary supplements can offer significant help before, during, and after cancer and cancer treatment.

TABLE 10-1

DIFFERENCES BETWEEN DRUGS
AND DIETARY SUPPLEMENTS

Drugs	Dietary supplements
Treat a pathology	Maintain well-being, wellness, and beauty
Used when a person is sick	Used when a person wants to remain healthy
Medically prescribed	Individually chosen to follow a healthier lifestyle
Therapeutic properties	Nutritional and physiological properties

"I'VE HAD CANCER": SUPPLEMENTS TO HELP YOU THROUGH

Let's start with the most simple, or if you prefer, the most urgent, situation. Let's talk first about which dietary supplements you can take if you have cancer or are in recovery—that is, they are not for cancer prevention. From experience, I know you will suffer from high stress, depression, loss of appetite, and tiredness, which is as much connected with the cancer as with its treatment, including surgery under anesthesia, radiation therapy, and chemotherapy. If you look at Table 10-2, you will see that I recommend you take ginseng, royal jelly, brewers' yeast, maca powder, wheat germ, camu camu (which is high in vitamin C, almost thirty to sixty times higher than oranges are), zinc, and magnesium. They will give your body both a physical and psychological boost. In fact, they will help you feel that you are taking active control of your illness, which explains why 70% of patients[4] who have had cancer take them. Also, to help your hair grow back after chemo-

TABLE 10-2

DIETARY SUPPLEMENTS TO TAKE DURING AND AFTER CANCER

Indication	My recommendations
Stress, tiredness, depression	Ginseng Royal jelly Brewers' yeast Maca powder Wheat germ Camu camu Zinc Magnesium
Hair growth	Brewers' yeast Vitamins B_1 and B_6
Weight loss	Green tea Caffeine Water-removing plants: common ash, meadowsweet

therapy, I recommend you take brewers' yeast and vitamin B_1 and B_6 supplements. Finally, to help you lose weight, so often gained during treatment, especially with certain molecules used with breast cancer, try green tea–based supplements, caffeine, and plants that deal with water retention (common ash, meadowsweet, etc.).

Always be prudent and ask your druggist for advice. Dietary supplements often contain a mixture of various substances, and some of them may have adverse interactions with your medication. Other undesirable effects are sometimes observed, like anticoagulation,[5] which is potentially dangerous if you have surgery scheduled. Moreover, some dietary supplements containing polyphenols might inhibit the elimination of drugs, thereby increasing their toxicity.[6]

Whatever your state of health, whatever your circumstances and requirements, I need to say: do not take any dietary supplements without giving it serious thought, and consult your oncologist first.

CAN DIETARY SUPPLEMENTS HELP PREVENT CANCERS, OR ARE THEY DANGEROUS?

Greater interest resides in dietary supplements because they may have the capacity to prevent certain cancers. Everything becomes far more complicated here, and the risks, in case of error, are much graver.

Contrary to what many believe, not all supplements help lessen our risk of getting cancer. Far from it! It has even been proved beyond doubt that some could do the exact opposite and actually promote the onset of certain cancers, including such serious cancers as lung cancer.

Let's begin with these dangerous supplements and with beta-carotene, a vitamin A derivative, the most dangerous one. Several studies have shown indisputably that beta-carotene considerably increases the risk of lung cancer in people who smoke or who have smoked. In most studies this risk increased by at least a third. The Beta-Carotene and Retinol Efficacy Trial (CARET),[7] carried out in the 1990s in the United States, included only men who smoked or had smoked in the past. The researchers stopped the trial prematurely when they realized that the risk of lung cancer in the group taking a 30-mg beta-carotene supplement daily was 28% higher than in the control group taking the placebo. The effect was even more marked in those who had been exposed to asbestos or who smoked very heavily.

CARET STUDY: BETA-CAROTENE AND RETINOL EFFICACY TRIAL

This American clinical trial was started in the early 1990s with eighteen thousand men who, being longtime smokers, were at a high risk of getting lung cancer. The study set out to measure the effect of daily beta-carotene supplementation on the incidence of lung cancers, other cancers, and cardiovascular diseases. Due to the increased incidence of lung cancers in the group taking beta-carotene supplements, the trial had to be stopped prematurely.

Four other studies[8-11] of the same type, including the ATBC study (see box below) looking at the effect of beta-carotene on the onset of lung cancer, reached the same conclusion: beta-carotene is harmful for our health and extremely dangerous for smokers or those who come into contact with tobacco smoke or any other substance that is potentially carcinogenic for our lungs (asbestos, hydrocarbon fumes, etc.).

ATBC STUDY: ALPHA-TOCOPHEROL BETA-CAROTENE CANCER PREVENTION STUDY

The ATBC study was carried out in Finland, between 1985 and 1993, on thirty thousand smokers. Its objective was to confirm the hypothesis that vitamin E and beta-carotene could protect against lung cancer. The results from the study showed an increased incidence of lung cancers in the group that had taken beta-carotene supplements.

This explains, incidentally, the reason why I recommend great caution in eating too much food particularly rich in beta-carotene for those people in the risk group.

In the French SUVIMAX cohort study, 13,017 adults, both men and women, were randomly selected. Half received a capsule every day containing vitamin C, vitamin E, beta-carotene, selenium, and zinc, and the other half received a placebo capsule. After the adults were monitored for more than seven years, a decrease in cancers was recorded in the men (but not in the women).[12] The researchers realized that a greater number of the men with high prostate-specific antigen (PSA) levels at the start of the study were developing prostate cancer,[13] and as with the previous study, more smokers were getting lung cancer and more women skin cancer.[14] It's all a little confusing!

SUVIMAX STUDY: ANTIOXIDANT VITAMIN AND MINERAL SUPPLEMENTATION

The SUVIMAX study was carried out for approximately eight years, starting in 1994 /1995, on a group of thirteen thousand volunteers. Its objective was to evaluate the impact of a nutritional dose of antioxidant vitamin and mineral supplementation on the incidence of cardiovascular and cancer pathologies and on mortality.

Another dietary supplement, retinol, produced nearly the same results.[15] This comes as no surprise since, like beta-carotene, retinol is a form of vitamin A. It must be avoided.

Vitamin E and iron

Vitamin E, or alpha-tocopherol, which the French happen to be particularly fond of, has turned out to be a real time-bomb as far as the risk of cancer is concerned. In 2008, the American National Cancer Institute stopped a large trial involving thirty-five thousand adults before it was due to end. The Selenium and Vitamin E Cancer Prevention Trial, or SELECT,[16] started in 2001. For this trial, the individuals who had volunteered were divided into four groups of approximately eight thousand each. The first group took selenium plus vitamin E; the second group, vitamin E only; the third, selenium only; and the fourth, a placebo. The study was stopped when the data showed that the supplements did not lower the incidence of prostate cancer and the subjects were told to stop taking them. In 2011, the researchers followed up with those in the study and found that the men who took vitamin E supplements had a 17% higher incidence of prostate cancer than those taking the placebo.[17]

SELECT STUDY: SELENIUM AND VITAMIN E CANCER PREVENTION TRIAL

The American clinical trial involving over thirty-five thousand men started in 2001 and had aimed to measure how effective selenium and/or vitamin E supplementation might be in preventing prostate cancer. The study showed a higher incidence of prostate cancer in men who had been given vitamin E supplements over those who were given the placebo.

As far as I am concerned, vitamin E should be avoided on principle, at least by men.

IN REGARD TO IRON, many studies have now proved that it increases the risk of colon cancer,[18] for both men and women, when compared to taking a placebo. Some studies have shown this risk to be three times greater. However, having said this, I would add that if someone has an iron deficiency, as is often the case with women suffering from very heavy periods, they obviously need to take extra iron.

DIETARY SUPPLEMENTS THAT DO YOU GOOD

Now let's take a look at dietary supplements that, fortunately for us, seem to have the effect of preventing cancer in humans.

Let's begin with selenium. One thing certain about selenium is that it protects against prostate cancer. Two recent studies[19, 20] have proved this beyond doubt. For example, in one study[21] of 974 people who had been selected because they had had a skin cancer (which I can assure you is totally irrelevant), seventeen cases of prostate cancer were recorded in the group taking selenium supplements, compared with thirty-five cases in the control group not getting supplements—that is, the incidence doubled. There are also indicators that as a dietary supplement, selenium might lower the risk of lung and colon cancer. To my mind, this is not at all bad for a product devoid of any real toxicity when taken in normal quantities. I would highly recommend it, at least in men over fifty.

Calcium is not bad either! In fact, a large number of studies have now proved that calcium supplementation reduces the risk of colorectal cancer by 20% to 25%.[22] This was shown after a total of 534,000 people were monitored during six to sixteen years. In accord with the World Cancer Research Fund report, I recommend this dietary supplement.

Moreover, three more recent major studies have proved that calcium supplementation significantly lowers (by 20% to 50%) the risk of the recurrence of polyps in the intestines,[23] which we know will become cancerous over time. This makes sense given that calcium has a preventive effect on colorectal cancer. So, if you have a colonoscopy and if one or more polyps are discovered, don't think twice about taking regular doses of calcium, after first seeking medical advice, of course.

And now for vitamin D!

Here, things get a little more complicated—mostly because I find it impossible to believe, as some affirm, that 42% of the American population[24] is deficient in vitamin D—in other words, that they don't have enough in their bodies.

How can 42% the American population, which overall enjoys good health, spends leisure time outdoors in the sun (the skin produces vitamin D when in contact with sunlight), and eats plenty of vitamin

D–rich food (dairy products, sardines, eggs, fish oils, and meats), have a deficiency of that vitamin? I think—once again, using the most elementary common sense—that the level of vitamin D stipulated as being normal must be set too high and thus a false number.

So what can we learn from the studies carried out on people? Twelve studies have looked at vitamin D supplementation and its impact on the risk of cancer, and, in particular, on colon cancer. Six of them showed a small decrease in risk, but it was too small to be considered significant. Two studies concluded that the risk of colon cancer was neither increased nor reduced by taking vitamin D, and four reached the conclusion that there was a slight increase in the risk of cancer, even if, once again, this increase was deemed too small to be considered significant.

As happens each time, a pooled analysis of all the studies came to the final conclusion that vitamin D supplementation had no impact on the risk of cancer, thus, it is unnecessary. However, and we discussed this when looking at dairy products, many studies that were not concerned with vitamin D as a dietary supplement, but rather with the role played by diets high in products containing vitamin D, concluded that these type of foods might play some small role in preventing colorectal cancer.[25] However, given that eating lots of dairy products increases the risk of prostate cancer[26] by almost 30%, we can recommend them for only women and children.

ANTICANCER NUTRIENTS

Alongside dietary supplements, there is another kind of substance many of you may take, thinking it might help prevent cancer: these are the nutrients. Certain of them are indeed of great interest.

Know that if you are particularly interested or would like to take part in trials in the United States on these products, information about all current trials is available on the National Institutes of Health website, at www.clinicaltrials.gov.

TABLE 10-3

**SOURCES, MECHANISMS OF ACTION, AND THE CANCERS ON WHICH
DIFFERENT NATURAL PROMOTER COMPONENTS WORK**[27]

Active substance	Natural source	Mechanism of action	Action on cancer types
Turmeric	Turmeric powder (*Curcuma longa*)	Antioxidant, anti-proliferation, anti-inflammation, anti-angiogenesis, immunomodulation	Skin, lung, oral cavity, head and neck, esophagus, stomach, liver, pancreas, small intestine, colon, bladder, prostate, mammary glands, lymphoma, cervix
Green tea (polyphenols, EGCG)	Green tea (*Camellia sinensis*)	Antioxidant, anti-mutagen, anti-proliferation, anti-inflammation, anti-angiogenesis, immunomodulation	Skin, lung, oral cavity, head and neck, esophagus, stomach, liver, pancreas, small intestine, colon, bladder, prostate, mammary glands
Luteolin	Artichokes, broccoli, celery, cabbage, spinach, green pepper, pomegranate leaf, peppermint, tamarind, cauliflower	Anti-inflammation, anti-allergy, anti-proliferation, antioxidant	Ovaries, stomach, liver, colon, breast, oral, adenocarcinoma of the esophagus, prostate, lung, nasopharynx, cervix, leukemia, skin, pancreas
Resveratrol	Red wine, grapes (especially the skin), blackberries, peanuts, vines, pine nuts	Antioxidant, anti-proliferation, anti-angiogenesis, anti-inflammation	Ovaries, breast, prostate, liver, womb, leukemia, lung, stomach
Genistein	Soy and soy products, red clover (*Trifolium pratense*), Sicilian pistachios (*Pistachia vera*)	Antioxidant, anti-proliferation, anti-angiogenesis, anti-inflammation	Prostate, breast, skin, colon, stomach, liver, ovaries, pancreas, esophagus, head and neck
Pomegranate	Pomegranates, pomegranate juice, pomegranate seed, pomegranate seed oil (*Punica granatum*)	Antioxidant, anti-proliferation, anti-angiogenesis, anti-inflammation	Prostate, skin, breast, lung, colon, oral, leukemia
Lycopene	Tomatoes, guava, rosehips, watermelons, papayas, apricots, pink grapefruit; especially abundant in red tomatoes and products made from tomatoes	Antioxidant, anti-proliferation, anti-angiogenesis, anti-inflammation, immunomodulation	Prostate, lung, breast, stomach, liver, pancreas, colorectal cancer, head and neck, skin

Table continues

Active substance	Natural source	Mechanism of action	Action on cancer types
Ellagic acid	Pomegranate juice, pomegranate seed oil, various nuts, edible honeysuckle (*Lonicera caurulea*), strawberries and other berries, Arjuna bark (*Terminalia arjuna*), belleric leaves and fruit (*Terminalia bellerica*) Muellers terminalia bark, leaves, and fruit (*Terminalia muelleri*)	Antioxidant, anti-proliferation, anti-inflammation	Neuroblastoma, skin, pancreas, breast, prostate, colon, intestine, esophagus, bladder, mouth, leukemia, liver
Lupeol	Mangoes, olives, figs, strawberries, red grapes	Antioxidant, anti-mutagenesis, anti-inflammation, anti-proliferation	Skin, lung, leukemia, pancreas, prostate, colon, liver, head and neck
Betulinic acid	Widely found in the plant kingdom; most prolific sources: birch tree (*Betula*), bear tree and other *Ziziphus* species, *Syzigium* species, *Diospyros* species (persimmon family), peony (*Paeonia* species)	Anti-inflammation, apoptosis, immunomodulation	Skin, ovaries, colon, brain, renal-cell carcinoma, womb, prostate, leukemia, lung, breast, head and neck
Ginkgolide B	*Ginkgo biloba*	Antioxidant, anti-angiogenesis	Ovaries, breast, brain

Turmeric

Turmeric, the first nutrient given in Table 10-3, is probably the most anticancerous. Taken from the roots of *Curcuma longa*, turmeric is a yellow pigment, very widely used as a spice. Interest in its medicinal properties has existed since ancient times. Recently it was shown that turmeric is capable of detoxifying carcinogenic substances, rendering them harmless, and does so by blocking the proliferation of many types of cancerous cells and driving them to suicide (apoptosis). Its impact is even more marked when combined with other nutrients such as genistein, green tea, embelin (a compound found in a type of Indian fruit), or the piperine in peppers. Turmeric enhances the effectiveness of many anticancer drugs used in chemotherapy. It has been tested in men to stop the reappearance of polyps in the colon; after six months of supplementation of turmeric combined with quercetin, the results have been very good. It can also be used to some effect as an ointment on malignant skin lesions. With regard to the prevention of particular cancers,[28] turmeric is clearly a nutrient with exciting potential.

Genistein

Genistein is a phytoestrogen found in plentiful supply in soy and bean sprouts. Here again, there seem to be many indicators that taking genistein might lower the risk of prostate, breast, and endometrial cancer. Genistein is thought to increase the effects of radiation therapy and to also work in synergy with some chemotherapy drugs. Like turmeric, it blocks cell division and drives cancerous cells to commit suicide.[29] At least two studies[30, 31] have shown genistein to be effective in slowing down the spread of prostate cancers and in delaying its recurrence.

Lycium barbarum **and other products**

Many substances are currently being tested on humans to see if they can prevent cancer. Among them is *Lycium barbarum*, a polysaccharide found in goji berries. By activating the p53 gene,[32] or "guardian of the genome," *L. barbarum* appears to be very powerful promoter of suicide in cancerous cells. It would seem to inhibit cell proliferation for many cancers, such as cancers of the prostate,[33] colon,[34] stomach,[35] breast,[36] and liver.[37] Even if it is still too early to confirm whether it can be used to prevent cancer, this is definitely a product to watch out for.

Other products are ellagic acid, lupeol, betulinic acid, luteolin, and the ones we have talked about elsewhere in this book, such as resveratrol, lycopene, pomegranate, polyphenols in green tea, and antho-cyanins in red berries.[38]

Going back to the old precepts of traditional medicines, these studies, both the in vitro ones and the ones on humans, are full of promise. However, prudence has led me to recommend in this book only the substances for which their positive effect on cancer prevention and the safety of their dosages have been shown in serious studies.

Chapter 11

....

Keeping Physically Active Keeps Us Healthy

....

We have now arrived at the last chapter before I give, as a closing, my anticancer advice. Although this chapter is not about a food group, there are good reasons to feature it in the book. More than once, while talking to you about meat, cheese, or foods containing sugar, fat, or a high-energy density, I have also spoken about cutting down your food intake, so that your weight will not go up year after year. It's time for me to address the problem of being overweight or obese, and to try to clarify the extraordinary development of this nutritional issue, which is becoming increasingly common in industrialized countries and elsewhere in the world. I will talk about the causes of too much weight gain and, more directly, its effect on specific cancers.

Unfortunately, being overweight or obese correlates with several types of cancer, including of the bladder, pancreas, colon, stomach, breast, kidney, endometrium, and esophagus. Obesity is thought to be directly responsible for 5% of these cancers.[1, 2]

WHY ARE WE GETTING SO FAT?

If you take a careful look at the body, and this is especially visible in children, you can see that it is built to move: it has 650 muscles and

TABLE 11-1

PREVALENCE OF OBESITY IN VARIOUS COUNTRIES IN 2010[3, 4]

Country	Prevalence (%)
United States	35.7
Canada	26
Great Britain	24
France	14
Brazil	12
Russia	10
China	4
Nigeria	3
India	2
Pakistan	2
Tanzania	1

214 bones, with tendons and joints that enable movement.[5] Can you think of all the movements your body is able to make? Our bodies are amazing feats of engineering, but we are putting them to less and less use.

We are no longer physically active. On the other side, living in our world of abundance, with food available 24/7, we are eating more and more high-fat or sugary foods all day long. Instead of providing fuel for physical exertion, these foods are accumulating passively in our fat cells as triglycerides, for example. We are becoming fatter, and our bodies are going by the wayside. That's the reason why we need to talk about physical activity and its effect on suppressing cancer.

However, before we go any further, what do we mean by obesity? Obesity is the most common nutritional problem. It is dependent on a variety of factors, such as lifestyle, sedentary behavior, eating habits, and psychological, genetic, and social determinants. We'll return to these causes a little later.

From 1997 on, the World Health Organization has defined being

TABLE 11-2

ENERGY USED FOR VARIOUS ACTIVITIES, IN CALORIES

Activity	Energy used (kcal/hour)
Sleeping, resting while sitting or lying down	60
Activities while sitting: watching TV, being on the computer, mealtimes, playing board games	90
Activities while standing up: getting ready in the morning, dressing, strolling	120
Women: exercising, gardening, walking, doing housework *Men*: average-intensity work while standing up	170
Men: gardening, high-intensity work	200
Sporting activities: skiing, swimming, jogging	> 300

overweight and obese as an abnormal or excessive accumulation of body fat that presents a risk to health.[6] A person is considered "overweight" when the fat cells (adipocytes) increase in size because more and more fat is being stored inside them. The term "obesity" is used when the fat cells reach saturation.

To define obesity accurately, we would need to precisely measure a person's body-fat mass and determine the level of it at which disease and mortality would increase for that person. Such calculations are far too complicated for a routine doctor's appointment. We use a simpler way of measuring obesity. Even though it does not allow us to pinpoint exactly where the fat is accumulating, which does have an effect on health, it does provide an indirect estimate of obesity.

The body mass index, or BMI, is used to calculate whether a person has a normal weight, is overweight, or is obese. It is based on the ratio of body mass (weight in pounds) divided by the square of the person's height (in inches). For example, the BMI for a woman who weighs 130 pounds and is 5 feet 4 inches tall is 22.3.

Adults with a BMI above 25 are considered overweight; those with a BMI above 30, obese (see Table 11-3). By using this measurement, we can study morbidity and mortality in direct relation to obesity.

TABLE 11-3

BMI CATEGORIES[7]

Category	BMI range
Underweight	< 18.5
Normal	18.5–24.9
Overweight	25.0–29.9
Moderate obesity	30.0–34.9
Severe obesity	35.0–39.9
Massive obesity	> 40.0

I bet you are already busy working out your own calculations. Wait until we have explained everything, so you can better understand why you've put on weight and you don't get too excited.

We must not forget that the risk from being overweight or obese also depends on age, on how the obesity developed, how long it has existed, and where the adipose tissue is distributed.

We also must not overlook the fact that children who are obese before the age of five will remain obese into adulthood. An analysis carried out by the National Center for Health statistics showed that in 2007–8, almost 17% of American children and teenagers were obese, with the highest percentage living in low-income households.

Low-income children and adolescents are more likely to be obese than their higher-income counterparts, but the relationship is not consistent across race and ethnicity groups.

Children and adolescents living in households where the head of the household has a college degree are less likely to be obese, compared with those living in households where the household head has less education, but the relationship is not consistent across race and ethnicity groups.[8]

THE UNITED STATES IS NOT alone in having increasing levels of obesity. In China, for example, where the population used to be known for being of smaller stature than Americans and being of normal weight, obesity levels have shot up in 2006, with 184 million Chinese overweight and 31 million obese.[9]

As you can see, obesity has developed into a dreadful affliction the world over. But you cannot simply get rid of a pathology like obesity as easily as you can shed a few surplus pounds. It is a complex phenomenon. In the body, when excess surplus energy is stored there is an initial phase with an increase in body-fat mass, after which point the body adapts to the new balance between energy input and output. It will then do everything it can to protect this new energy balance and keep the fat.

You may be asking the same question I did: "But how come we've become too fat?" Is the American way of life, meaning being addicted to video games, eating take-out food at all times of the day and night, and buying ready-made food (see Table 11-4) made entirely from fats and sugars, responsible for that?

According to scientists, clinicians, and epidemiologists, the reasons are manifold but debatable.

Some studies have talked about the role of the food industry, which produces foods with a very high glycemic index.[10] Such foods are packed with corn syrup, full of fructose. Studies have also looked at the part played by fast-food outlets and vending machines selling candy in schools.[11]

But let's not get carried away. These studies have not proved that these eating habits are to blame for the increase in BMI.

TABLE 11-4

CHANGES IN AVERAGE ANNUAL INTAKE BETWEEN 1970–79 AND 2000[12, 13]

	Change
Fruit juices	+ 9%
Sweetened beverages	+ 135%
Total grain products	+ 44%
Rice, milled	+ 170%

Although it detected connections between obesity and eating fast-food, the Burdette and Whitaker study[14] cannot claim to link cause with effect. Sugary drinks like sodas seem to provide the most convincing lead and the closest link to obesity and a high BMI. At any rate, this is the result from three of four studies carried out on American children.[15]

Other studies have mentioned the time spent in front of the television, snacking on high-energy foods (potato chips, junk food, etc.). A recent meta-analysis concluded that there is a statistical link but insufficient clinical proof to confirm it.[16] These studies are not questioning the importance of these factors; they are saying that further possibilities need to be considered as well.

Lack of sleep is mentioned in other scientific arguments. For both children and adults, a significant amount of time spent sleeping decreases the risk of a high BMI and the risk of obesity.[17]

How do we work out what is going on? How do we decide what's the cause? As you can see, there is a whole range of reasons for this increase in obesity. Whenever obesity is mentioned, we never talk about a single cause. However, the epidemiological studies and plausible mechanisms for these causes have not yet been sufficiently substantiated. Even if the repercussions, stemming from one of the causes, are only minor, all these causes when combined may have truly far-reaching consequences for obesity.

But why should being overweight be a factor that promotes cancer? The reason is that extra fat adds to the conditions that alter several biochemical parameters directly involved in the metabolism of cancerous cells.

We won't reexamine in close detail the mechanisms that lead to an increased risk of cancer for the overweight or obese. We looked at this in the chapter about sugars and sugary products. Let's just say that these adipocytes behave like true hormone pumps. They stimulate secretion of insulin, a hormone that controls our metabolism of energy, the use and storage of sugar. Surplus insulin can stimulate cell proliferation, including of cancerous cells. It does so either by acting directly on the cancerous cells or by stimulating the liver to secrete another hormone, insulin-like growth factor (IGF), which is also a very powerful cancer-promoting factor. Finally, both insulin and IGF1 have an unfortunate tendency to boost the activity of the enzymes in our body that produce the sexual hormones estradiol in women and testosterone in men. A consequence of an increase in the proliferation of these cells in a woman's breasts or a man's prostate is, therefore, an elevated risk of developing breast or prostate cancer.

PHYSICAL ACTIVITY PLAYS A PREVENTIVE ROLE

What then is the direct connection between obesity, physical activity, and cancer?

We have just seen the connection between obesity and cancer. Let's carry on by looking at the role physical activity plays, because it too is crucial in stopping the promotion of certain cancers. The way we are able to increase or decrease the amount of energy we burn is basically through varying the amount of physical activity we do. The more physically active we are, the less sugars and lipids remain available to turn into triglycerides (fats) in our adipocytes. Are you starting to make the connection? Remember, the equation is very simple:

Energy stored = Energy taken in – Energy used

Apart from life-supporting physical activity, we use energy for:

- thermoregulation, the energy process that enables us to keep our bodies at a constant temperature of around 98.6° F, regardless of how hot or cold it is around us;
- and basic metabolism, another energy process that allows us to keep all our vital functions in good working order. We need more or less energy depending on whether we are slim, fat, a heavy smoker, male, female, and so on.

Physical activity, along with making you lose weight, can influence the inhibition of cancers. When we exercise, the muscles contract so that the body can move, and this contraction requires energy. To release this energy, the muscle has to use up endogenous (already stored in the body) glucose or exogenous sugars, which come directly from what we eat and drink. The more intense the muscular contraction and the longer it lasts, the more carbohydrates get used. This is an efficient way of using the sugars and lipids we ingest. If we don't do any exercise, the sugars and lipids will otherwise get stored in the body, filling up our adipocytes.

The respective contributions from the burning of carbohydrates (fast release) or lipids (slower release) to supply energy vary according to the intensity of the exercise, the nutritional status, and the physical capacity of the individuals being studied.

How does this work?

Physical activity affects the body in the way it makes the body draw from its energy reserves, stored away unutilized in its fat cells, and curbs the cancer-promoting factors that we just discussed. You see, exercise work's on the body's interaction with what we consume, and as I told you, that can help offset the effects of a diet where the calorie intake is too high.

We know so much about the influence physical activity has on cancer because cancer specialists and numerous scientists have scientifically tested and measured the impact physical activity has on men and women with endometrial, breast, prostate, or colon cancer, and these broad studies have proved the positive effects of physical activity against cancer.[18-22] In 2008, the United States Cochrane Institute published twenty-eight studies proving that physical activity increases the likelihood of surviving cancer; sixteen of them were for breast cancer.[23]

As well as improving the quality of life (the thrust of three essays published in 2008)[24]—along with self-esteem, tiredness, and tolerance of treatments—physical activity can sometimes improve the chances of recovery.

WHAT PHYSICAL ACTIVITY IS ANTICANCER?

As well as having an influence on cancer once it has become established, physical activity may also have a prophylactic effect by acting on the factors connected with weight problems that are cancer promoters. Physical activity alters estrogen metabolism and boosts the production of low-estrogen derivatives. It lowers insulin levels and insulin resistance in sedentary and overweight women, as many studies have shown. One study on long-term overweight women being treated for cancer confirmed that appropriate physical activity, in itself, has a truly positive impact.[25–28]

If you want to exercise and at the same time protect yourself against the onset of cancer, the type of physical activity you choose has to follow a specific protocol.[29, 30] Energy expended must be worked out in MET (metabolic equivalent of task) hours and not in kilocalories. One MET hour is an estimate of how much oxygen a person uses when remaining at rest for one hour. That amount corresponds to 3.5 mL of O_2 per kilogram per minute.

Walking, for example, is equivalent to 3 MET hours. If you walk at a brisk pace or go upstairs, that can border on 6 MET hours. Strenuous exercise such as jogging, tennis, or swimming will add up to more than 6 MET hours (see Table 11-5). A 2011 study from the Centers for Disease Control and Prevention showed that only 20.6% of adults get the required amount of aerobic muscle-strengthening activity.[31] I imagine that this figure will help you understand just how sedentary we have become!

For physical activity to have an impact on the prognosis of postmenopausal women with cancer, their weekly exercise has to be equivalent to 9 MET hours, for example, three 1-hour walks per week, or 1 hour of swimming and 30 minutes of walking per week, or 30 minutes of walking six times a week. Three studies arrived at this same conclusion: the American Nurses' Health Study, with 2,987 patients[32] the Women's Healthy Eating and Living (WHEL) study, with 1,490 patients[33] and the Collaborative Women's Longevity Study (CWLS), with 4,482 participants.[34]

TABLE 11-5

ESTIMATED ENERGY EXPENDITURE FOR VARIOUS ACTIVITIES[35]

Sporting activities	MET hours	Everyday living	MET hours
Yoga	2.5–3.5	Sitting	1
Aqua aerobics	4	Cooking	2
Jogging in the gym	4.5	Housework	2–4
Cycling	4–10	DIY	3–5
Rowing	3.5–6.5	Walking	2–3
Swimming	4–11	Gardening	3–6
Tennis	5–8		
Martial Arts	10		
Squash	12		

Note: DIY, do-it-yourself jobs.

As far as colon cancer is concerned, energy expenditure needs to be 18 MET, greater than what was studied for breast cancer, as shown in the Cancer and Leukemia Group B (CALGB) study.[36]

Used prophylactically after a cancer, physical exercise must be for both the legs and the arms, include resistance training, and last for at least thirty minutes. Unfortunately, if your BMI is above 30, the preventative effects of physical activity will be less, so try to keep your BMI under 30.

Don't hesitate any longer: you absolutely must include some physical activity in your daily routine. Walk for at least thirty minutes every day; take up a sport such as tennis, swimming, or gymnastics; garden or do some heavy housework. Housekeeping also helps burn energy.

Educate your children about sports. Cancer risk can be reduced by physical activity between the ages of twelve and twenty-two.

If you are overweight, try to combine eating a more balanced diet with doing regular, moderate exercise.

I could just stop here with my recommendations, but this wouldn't be quite fair. If you aren't exercising or never have exercised, there has to be a good reason why.

Since the alarming upsurge in obesity, gyms, which started to become popular in the mid-1980s, changed their marketing slogans. Around 1995 there was a shift from the social reasons for having a beautiful body, which was a symbol of success, to the physical reasons to have a healthy body, which was as important as psychological health. This was the birth of "wellness," as opposed to "fitness," which is more concerned with having a body that is aesthetically beautiful rather than meeting health parameters.

You are told, "Exercise, it's good for your health." You are overwhelmed with a menu of activities, with names that are increasingly more outrageous: hi-low, step, body pump, and so on. But which one should you choose? With such an abundance of exercises available, it is very important to find an activity in keeping with who you are. How can you really do yourself some good? How can you make being physically active a necessary part of your lifestyle and necessary to your well-being? It is well known that a physical activity that is not right for you has little chance of motivating you.

In such a case, you will find no pleasure in doing this exercise and will probably give it up quickly, having spent a tidy sum and feeling guilty deep-down.

Pick an activity that reflects your deeper aspirations, emotions, interests, and affinities, as well as how you manage stress, your ability to adapt, and your concentration. The way you decide to be physically active is also about the way you decide to express yourself and who you are.

If you are not especially competitive, what is the point in taking up tennis? How could you enjoy yoga if you have no interest in introspection? Why get involved with team sports if you are of a more solitary temperament and more inclined toward individual sports? So telling you to "try this sport or activity because it's the best one for your health" is very arbitrary. It would be the equivalent of making you eat the broccoli that you hate, when you'd rather be diving into the cauliflower that you love.

Although meditation and relaxation will help you manage your stress levels, these activities do not "burn off enough energy" to have an impact on the physiological parameters that trigger the onset of cancers. As we have seen, to tackle weight problems and their cancer-related downsides, you will need to do aerobic exercise. Your exercise needs to involve cardiorespiratory effort equivalent to at least 60% of your maximum heart rate (pulse), which is calculated as "220 – your age." Also, you need to burn energy equivalent to at least 3 MET hours. I have not forgotten that you might be a little or even quite significantly overweight and that this doesn't make the task any easier. You tire more quickly, your weight hinders your movements, and your joints have a lot of pressure to bear.

ECOLOGYMS

I'm going to therefore suggest that you try what I call "ecologyms."

Let's use your car as an example. You are told that you need to find a way of getting it to work perfectly, using less polluting fuel while not putting it under strain. This would be a good way of making your car last longer and be safer to drive.

Ecologyms follow exactly the same principle, but for your body. The aim is to exert yourself, but to protect your body—to exercise in a way that is not too harsh on your body, but that also lets you burn off sufficient energy.

Ecologyms often involve fluid movements that enable better circulation of energy and improved coordination; unstable positions that require a good knowledge of the body and a refinement of balance, which increases our capacity for concentration; and, finally, deep breathing, which helps to slow down the heart and, in turn, alleviates stress.

All you have to do now is bear this in mind. Remember that it is essential to find the discipline and type of movement that fits who you are and will allow your body to express itself with joy.

THESE ARE THE "ECOLOGYMS" I suggest you try:

- **Water aerobics.** This is gymnastics done in the water, where you are immersed (for most of the exercises) in the water up to your shoulders. I advise you to try aqua aerobics if you are overweight, because the body weighs less in the water and the resistance from the water intensifies the exercises. It is also easier on the joints.
- **Hiking.** Walking with a group of people in a natural environment is an excellent way of doing moderate physical exercise without realizing you're even doing it, since you become so focused on the walk and your surroundings. Using a stick in each hand, as with Nordic walking, makes it more strenuous.
- **Stretching.** Stretching helps improve flexibility in all muscle groups while focusing on breathing in deeply. It's ideal if you suffer from muscular tension and need to relax.
- **Pilates.** Although it has been around since the early twentieth century when Joseph Pilates invented it, Pilates has now become very popular. Using roller/pulley machines, the aim is to get the body to adopt positions with perfect posture and alignment. It is an excellent method for strengthening the deep abdominal muscles and for the body to regain balance, posture, and flexibility.
- **Tai Chi and Qigong.** The great advantage of these Asian disciplines is the fluidity of their gestures, which require great balance and concentration, with rhythmic deep breathing. Both are very relaxing. Nowadays sessions are organized outdoors in parks and public gardens.
- **Power yoga.** This has become very popular in recent years. It is a very physical type of yoga that works with sequences of yoga positions. It helps make physical and psychological stress fall away.

Each of these activities will foster your wish to exercise on your own, to be playful, or to be creative. You are bound to find one that you really enjoy and that will help you take up physical exercise again, or for the first time, but without it feeling like a real chore. Without even thinking about it, you'll add to your repertoire a genuine cancer-prevention program.

Chapter 12

·····················

Anticancer Advice

···

You now know everything, or just about everything, about most foods: what they contain, good or ill, their virtues and the dangers they occasionally present. You have probably formed some idea of what you now intend to eat more of and, possibly too, what you will cut out of your diet or, at any rate, what you will eat less of.

So far so good.

But, along with Nathalie Hutter-Lardeau, the nutritionist who has given me much help in writing this book, I think it's preferable to give you some nutritional advice to optimize your anticancer standpoint, rather than making you figure out conclusions on your own from all you've read. We have tried to put all the major information about foods into perspective, showing how they coordinate their actions, and how to compensate for their failings, so you can draw the greatest possible advantages from this new science of nutrigenomics, which has helped us understand the role played by food in the development of a cancer.

Now here is what we have called our "anticancer advice."

FIVE GOLDEN RULES

However, before examining this advice in detail, I want to start off by giving you the Five Golden Rules. In reality, no matter how you change your diet, you will be unable to significantly lower your risk of cancer without them. Here are the Five Golden Rules. They are extremely simple:

1. **Don't smoke.** Although we have seen that a first glass of wine is not carcinogenic, smoking is positively carcinogenic from the very first cigarette. This may also be the case for secondhand smoke, that is, when someone nearby is smoking. So, whatever happens, don't smoke and, most importantly, make sure that your children don't smoke either, especially when they are young.

2. **Eat a varied diet.** Don't deprive yourself of anything, even if, from time to time, you want to indulge yourself by eating something that might be dangerous for your health. When we talk about dangerous carcinogenic effects, we are actually talking about eating a significant amount of a specific food regularly over a long period of time. If, for example, you enjoy salmon and some salmon are full of heavy metals, you are not going to develop a cancer because you consume an 8-oz. (200-g) portion of this fish every once in a while.

3. **Vary how you cook your food.** It is true that cooking with a wok is potentially carcinogenic. It is also true that when organic substances, which would mean all foods, come into contact with flames—in other words, are cooked at very high temperatures—highly carcinogenic substances appear in the smoke around the person who is cooking, as well as on and inside the food itself.

   From this point of view, steaming or stewing food is far better for one's health. It is also true, for reasons we have already examined, that frying food may be harmful. However, despite this, there is nothing to stop you from having a couple of barbecues in the summer or from occasionally eating Asian food. Or even from making yourself a portion of French fries, especially if, instead of drowning them in oil, you use one of the new appliances that allow you to make a couple of pounds with just a spoonful of oil.

4. **Choose to eat products that are made by hand, locally produced, and farmed by sustainable (or sound) methods.** We
   have seen how the idea of local foods is important. My
   friend Jean Luc Petitrenaud, a prestigious French journalist
   specializing in gastronomy, has told me that often! We have
   seen how the idea of terroir has guaranteed us high-quality
   products for which recipes or production methods have
   been passed down through time and history, across a
   region and a people. We have seen how local foods have
   generally proved to be relatively innocuous for health and
   sometimes even of benefit in preventing certain illnesses.

   Even if eating "organic food" has never been scientifically proved to be beneficial as regards to the risk of cancer,
   always opt for products grown with the least amount of
   pesticides, either organic products (unfortunately, they are
   often expensive) or ones produced through sustainable
   farming. Wash your food, and don't hesitate, whenever
   possible, to give it an initial wash with some slightly soapy
   water, the better for removing residual pesticides, and then
   rinse it thoroughly before eating.

5. **Fix your energy balance.** Try to increase the amount you
   exercise and reduce the amount of calories you consume.
   Make sure you have an appropriate body mass index. Do
   not eat too many rich foods, which means you'll need to
   pay attention to the fats and sugars hidden in certain
   foods. Do not snack between meals. Do exercise. And if
   one day you feel like celebrating and you really want to
   indulge yourself, then go ahead. But, afterward, spend one
   or two days on a low-calorie diet to make up for it and run
   an extra half mile so that you also feel less guilty.

You should know that Laënnec, one of the most renowned French
physicians of the eighteenth century, had a habit of saying that diseases were the result of sad feelings. So, don't be sad! Eat happily, and
whatever in theory the ramifications might be, don't stop yourself from
enjoying a little indulgence as long as it is only once in a while.

These are, to my mind, the ground rules that form the foundation on which we can lay down our anticancer advice for you. But, first, I think that some of you might like a table that recapitulates the antioxidant power of the main foods we have talked about in this book.

However, as we have seen, for example, with beta-carotene and vitamin E—two powerful antioxidants—I warn you against the too widespread idea that what is good for preventing cancer essentially consists of eating antioxidants.

TABLE 12-1

ANTIOXIDANT CONTENT IN DIFFERENT FOODS[1]

Food	Number of samples analyzed	Antioxidant content (mmol/100 g)
DRINKS	283	8.3
Black tea, ready to drink	5	1
Milky hot chocolate	4	0.4
Coffee, made with a filter and boiled	31	2.5
Espresso, ready to drink	2	14.2
Green tea, ready to drink	17	1.5
Red wine	27	2.5
BREAKFAST BREADS	90	1.1
White bread, toasted	3	0.6
Whole-wheat bread, toasted	2	1
FRUIT AND FRUIT JUICES	278	1.25
Apples	15	0.4
Dried apricots	4	3.1
Dried apples	3	3.8
Dried blueberries	1	48.3
Dried dates	2	1.7
Dried mangoes	2	1.7
Oranges	3	0.9
Papayas	2	0.6
Prunes	1	3.2
Pomegranates	6	1.8
Strawberries	4	2.1

Apple juice	11	0.3
Cranberry juice	5	0.92
Grape juice	6	1.2
Orange juice	16	0.6
Pomegranate juice	2	2.1
Prune juice	3	1
Tomato juice	14	0.48
CEREALS AND CEREALS PRODUCTS	227	0.34
Barley	4	1
Whole-wheat bread	3	0.5
Light buckwheat flour	2	1.4
Dark buckwheat flour	2	2
Cornmeal	3	0.6
Millet	1	1.3
VEGETABLES	69	0.48
Artichokes	8	3.5
Peas	25	0.8
Black olives	6	1.7
Cooked broccoli	4	0.5
Red and green chilis	3	2.4
Kale	4	2.8
NUTS AND SEEDS	90	4.57
Hazelnuts	1	4.7
Roasted peanuts	1	2
Pecans	7	8.5
Pistachios	7	1.7
Sunflower seeds	2	6.4
Walnuts	13	22
SPICES AND HERBS	425	29
Dried basil	5	19.9
Dried coriander	3	26.5
Cloves	6	277
Dried dill	3	20
Dried tarragon	3	43.8

(Table continues)

Food	Number of samples analyzed	Antioxidant content (mmol/100 g)
SPICES AND HERBS	425	29
Ginger	5	20.3
Dried mint leaves	2	116
Dried oregano	9	63.2
Dried bay leaves	5	44.8
Saffron	3	44.5
Thyme	3	56.3
FOODS OF ANIMAL ORIGIN	211	0.18
Dairy products	86	0.14
Eggs	12	0.04
Fish and products from the sea	32	0.11
Meat and meat-based products	31	0.31
Poultry and poultry-based products	50	0.23

OUR ANTICANCER ADVICE

It seems to me that one good way to begin is by giving you two important lists: a list of what you ought to generally avoid, and a list of what you should try to eat.

Anticancer agents

Let's start off with the top-ten good things:

1. **Pomegranate juice.** Processed pomegranate juice is even better for your health because it is richer in very-high-quality antioxidants.
2. **Turmeric.** Don't hold back; put it in everything. It is one of the most powerful anticancer supplements.
3. **Green tea.** All types of green tea are packed with epigallocatechin-3-gallate and are excellent, especially, so it seems, when combined with dried, papaya-leaf tea.

4. **Wine.** Red wine is full of resveratrol. You can drink it in small quantities, on average two (women) to three (men) glasses a day.

5. **Selenium.** One of the few supplements that have been shown to be effective in preventing cancer, selenium is widely available at drugstores. Ask your doctor or druggist for advice.

6. **Tomatoes.** These are particularly good when eaten as commercially produced tomato sauces and tomato juice. They contain lycopene, which offers great protection against cancer, especially in men.

7. **Dietary fiber.** Dietary fiber is very important not only as prebiotics but also because, when undigested, it goes more quickly through the intestinal transit and thus reduces the time the mucus membranes are in contact with any potentially carcinogenic products in the food. However, anyone with irritable-bowel syndrome should exercise caution.

8. **Garlic and onions.** These remarkable anticancer agents also play a huge part in the famous Mediterranean diet. Whenever you can, add them to your food.

9. **Quercetin.** Found particularly in capers, lovage, cocoa, and hot chili peppers, quercetin is excellent cancer-prevention agent, especially for smokers.

10. **Physical exercise.** This plays a major role in reducing the risk of cancer recurrence. Exercise also directly ensures that we expend enough energy to keep our body mass index at a satisfactory level.

These are the best anticancer agents available at our disposition. They are easy to use or do, and not just for the elite; at a modest cost they are available to everyone. They form the base, the central core of the anticancer advice I want to give you. They are the least open to question and the most scientifically accepted. More generally, with these top-ten suggestions you can act now to try to lower your personal risk for developing a cancer—as far as that is possible, of course.

Along with this list, I consider it quite sensible to give you another one, but this time for the "flop ten." These are the ten things you should avoid in your daily life if you have decided to take your health in hand and are trying to reduce your chances of getting cancer.

What you should avoid

Let's go through this list together.

1. **Smoking.** I am sorry, but I cannot help mentioning this again. Don't forget that smoking alone is responsible for almost 30% of all cancers in the United States.

Fine, but since including smoking on this list is cheating slightly, I am going to start counting from one again.

1. **An excess of swordfish, red tuna, halibut, and salmon.** These fish contain too many toxic heavy metals for you to eat them often. At any rate, avoid eating them on a daily basis.
2. **An excess of dairy products, both milk and fermented products (cheese, yogurt) for men.** After the age of fifty, men should not eat much of them. However, for women and children, these products are excellent.
3. **Beta-carotene.** This is found in many of the food supplements sold in drugstores and on the Internet. Please take note: if you smoke, or if you used to smoke, please avoid beta-carotene as it is very harmful to your health. Be careful, too, if you tend to eat large quantities of fruits and vegetables containing beta-carotene. The same goes for vitamin A and other derivatives such as retinoids.
4. **Vitamin E.** There was a time when vitamin E was highly recommended. As it happens, we ought to be very careful with this vitamin as it has now been proved to increase the risk of certain cancers. Here again, exercise caution, as vitamin E is found in lots of vitamin cocktails, sold both in

drugstores as well as on the Internet. Once again, don't meddle with this dangerous substance.

5. **An excess of alcohol.** A little from time to time probably does no harm, but when consumed on a regular basis, alcohol can lead to a greater risk for certain cancers.

6. **Excessive weight.** Watch out, you can't ignore this any longer. Just as a sedentary lifestyle is a powerful factor for cancer risk, so is being overweight. The best thing men and women can do is to pay attention to their weight, and to do this from an early age, for themselves and their children.

7. **Arsenic in drinking water, and nitrites and nitrates in water and in some commercially produced meat products.** Routinely avoid arsenic, nitrites, and nitrates as they are highly carcinogenic. Check to see if there are any in your tap water. Read the labels on commercial sausages and delicatessen meats.

8. **Blood in meat.** Get rid of blood in meat by, for example, rinsing the meat before you prepare it. If, as a treat, you have a meal of a lightly cooked hamburger along with a juicy rib of beef, take a calcium phosphate tablet afterward. Very well-respected French researchers say that this should reduce the potentially carcinogenic effect of the hemoglobin found in the blood you eat.

9. **Fats high in polyunsaturated fatty acids.** In particular avoid rapeseed, perilla, and hempseed oils. As far as the risk of cancer is concerned, they seem to be potentially dangerous, especially at a very high temperature.

10. **Grilling food and cooking with a wok.** Do not cook with a wok, especially if you also use the oils we just listed. When any food gets burnt by coming into contact with flames (> 500°C or 932°F), it creates particularly harmful substances. The same happens when cooking with a wok, the very shape of which can lead to much-too-high cooking temperatures, which will produce carcinogenic products.

Now we have taken a tour of the main things that are potentially harmful for our health, concerning the risk of cancer.

Fasting

I should mention fasting, which has been practiced since the dawn of time, often in accordance with religious or philosophical beliefs. For animals in a laboratory, fasting has at times, reduced the risk of cancer. It seems that the production of ketonic bodies, which arise during fasting or carbohydrate-free dieting, could make cancer cells—unlike healthy cells—fragile or disable their metabolism from functioning. Equally, there may be a drop in the secretion of some growth factors capable of stimulating cell multiplication, such as IGF1, as we have seen. I cannot recommend that you try fasting, but I thought that I should mention it now. Especially if you have or have had cancer, you should not fast; it is certain that fasting will weaken you. I consider long fasts to be absolutely forbidden for anyone in such circumstances, especially when in the course of cancer treatment or when weak.

A few tips on eating fruits and vegetables

Several times throughout this book we talked about fruits and vegetables, and for the most part they are marvelous anticancer agents.

However, we did mention one note of caution: malignant melanoma might be linked to drinking too much orange juice, especially for those exposed to the sun or at risk from melanoma (however, further studies are needed to confirm this very recent claim).

It seems important in this chapter of anticancer advice to recommend to you the optimal way to eat these foods. Might we be able to do this according to their colors? This is how we proceeded in the chapter where we discussed them. Of course, it may seem that for the first time in this book we are venturing into clearly less scientific territory, but I believe nevertheless that choosing fruits and vegetables by color contains a certain logic if you are familiar with how these foods work and the molecular targets on which they are acting.

As a general rule, it is better to eat orange or orange-yellow fruit and vegetables in the morning, when their antioxidant properties can repair the damage from the night before. Green fruit and vegetables are more for the evening, as they get their color from photosynthesis connected with the sun's activity. It is certainly best to avoid purple or dark-colored fruit and vegetables in the evening, because they are often acidic.

Red and white fruits and vegetables can be eaten all day long, whenever you wish, without any restrictions.

Advice to fit every age

I also believe that there is specific dietary advice appropriate to age, gender, and smokers—for the first group, because of the extremely carcinogenic effect of female hormones; for the next group, because of the very particular risks connected with prostate cancer; and for the last one, because the number of lesions and therefore of repairs necessary to keep a smoker's genetic material in good order is considerably higher than for a non-smoker.

So here are few extra pieces of advice for people in these different groupings.

1. **Premenopausal women.** Women who are premenopausal are full of female hormones that, even though beneficial in many ways, are nonetheless dangerous for the breasts and uterus. At this age, although there is already a considerable risk of breast cancer, what is of most significance is that these women are starting to produce lesions in their mammary cells which could lead to breast cancers that will, for the majority, be detected after menopause.

   It is important for premenopausal women to exercise and to keep a very strict eye on their weight. They need to eat copious amounts of dairy products and take calcium supplements. After giving birth, they should breastfeed. Selenium is very good too. They should opt for low-alcohol wines (drinking in moderation, in any case), and they must give up smoking. For them, green and white fruits and vegetables are best. Fiber is also very important, since in recent years there has been an increase in the number of cases of colon cancer in women. The risk will soon be as great for women as it is for men, and this is perhaps linked to the fact that women are eating less and less fiber. Bread, especially brown or whole-wheat bread, is excellent to eat. At this age, women run the risk of iron deficiency because of menstruation. Even if, as we have seen, iron can be dangerous, they must not be deficient in it. Therefore, it is necessary for premenopausal women to eat red meat, lentils, green beans, tofu, chickpeas, figs, and apricots, especially if they have very heavy periods. They may also take vitamin C supplements, which increase absorption of iron in the stomach. At this age, the need for orange fruit and vegetables is limited, especially for women who smoke.

A word, here, regarding deodorants, especially after we advised you to regularly exercise: A completely ridiculous idea has been circulating everywhere that deodorants cause breast cancer by having a local effect. How preposterous! I'm not even going to examine in detail the biomolecular explanations that would prove this to be mere nonsense and rubbish. I will just remind you that we usually apply deodorant to both armpits, under both arms. If it were true that deodorants have a carcinogenic effect on the breast near the armpit, women ought to have cancers in both breasts. However, bilateral breast cancer is very rare, indeed, even extremely rare if we leave out the women who carry the hereditary BRCA gene and who, regardless of any deodorant issues, tend to have bilateral breast cancer during their lifetime. And what about breast cancer in men, who also use deodorants? Male breast cancer is virtually unheard of. Let's put a stop to such stupid ideas. You may use deodorants under your arms. Don't return, I beg you, to the odors of the Middle Ages.

2. **Postmenopausal women**. For these women, calcium and selenium are vital. If you fall into this category, ask your druggist for advice. Iron is not good, so avoid it. As a rule, fats are harmful for you, especially those high in polyunsaturated fatty acids. If you eat foods full of toxic products, such as some types of fish, then have fiber as part of the same meal to speed along your digestion. Eat lots of fruits and vegetables, especially ones that are green, white, and dark-colored. Drink green tea and eat ginger (and why not combine them?), as well as capers, cocoa, lovage, and hot chili peppers.

   Of course, continue doing regular exercise, and keep an eye on your body mass index, which really must remain below 25.

3. **Men.** Men who smoke should avoid beta-carotene. This is absolutely essential.

   Otherwise, whether they smoke or not, men must make sure that they take in as little vitamin E and calcium as possible. They should restrict their intake of dairy products. If they have a meal with a lot of cheese, they should eat a "scavenger" food containing fiber, for example, a banana or green tea. They should eat as much red fruit and vegetables as possible, especially tomatoes. It is best not to eat fresh tomatoes, but processed ones, like tomato sauce, which contain far more lycopene. If you are fair-haired, stop drinking orange juice and try pomegranate juice instead. Eat as much white fruits and vegetables as you can; garlic, onions, spring onions, and shallots are excellent for your health.

   Selenium is also very good for you. Go see your doctor or pharmacist. Eat pulses (peas and beans). Avoid blood in red meat. Drink wine in moderation, without exceeding an average of three glasses a day. And give up smoking, as it is the most dangerous thing you can do.

Avoid all multivitamin tablets that contain retinol or one of its derivatives. Be careful drinking water; check that it does not contain arsenic. Anything containing quercetin is good for you (capers, cocoa, lovage, and hot chili peppers).

Exercise and watch your weight. Do not let your body mass index exceed 25.

Avoid grilled meats and processed deli meats.

Voilà, we have summarized some anticancer advice that I think is useful for you, and a little more personalized than what you are normally offered. Of course, this advice does not in any way contradict or rule out the Five Golden Rules listed at the start of the chapter or the recommendations concerning what is good ("top ten," page 199) and bad (flop ten, page 200) for you.

The information specified by age, gender, and smoking status completes and personalizes the general lists. All in all, it will enable you to think better about what is good for you and, as far as is possible, to lower your risk of developing a cancer during your lifetime.

However, as we will see in the conclusion that follows, we do not claim that our dietary recommendation will radically change your risk of cancers, or eliminate it or reduce it to zero, or even, more simply, lower it by 50% or more, as some others have claimed for their diets. No, more modestly but also more scientifically and truthfully, our advice will enable you to score a few points as you fight cancer, that dreadful scourge. In so doing, you can slightly increase your chances of avoiding it or of avoiding a relapse by taking preventive measures.

Following this advice should not in any way tempt you to stop taking part in cancer-screening programs. When I was chairman of the French National Cancer Institute (INCA), I battled against all the odds to ensure that my fellow citizens could enjoy equal access to screening programs for cervical, breast, skin, and colon cancer. Let me assure you that these screening tests are effective and can lower your risk of cancer, or at any rate of serious cancer—so please take advantage of them.

Conclusion

....

Now I believe I have told you everything, explained everything, and commented on everything. If you have read these pages carefully, you now know everything, or close to everything, there is to know about the links between nutrition and cancer.

I have tried, throughout all the chapters, with the greatest honesty possible, to simplify this information and make it comprehensible to you. What is more, I have tried to do this in such a way that you can draw your own conclusions about the best way to eat, at least as far as the risk of cancer is concerned.

For me, writing this book has been an exciting journey into the scientific fields of nutrition and nutrigenomics. I have learned some unexpected and fascinating things that have often shaken my certainties and beliefs as a consumer.

In order to simplify the data, I have had to read, understand, and digest many hundreds of articles. I have held discussions with dozens of specialists and researched a very large number of websites. However, the plus side at the end of this Herculean task is that I have been able to create a health project that I hope will be as useful for you as it was for me. I wrote it, not only to put all the possible chances on our side and to try to lower our risk of developing a cancer—may I remind you that in the United States almost one in two men and almost one in three women will be affected by cancer in their lifetime—but also to try to protect our children and grandchildren from cancer as far as possible, because that is an area where much remains to be done.[1]

I have shown what could lessen your risk of cancer, and I have pointed out what could increase it. I have dared to reveal the truth about foods or their quality, showing them to be up for debate, and about some dietary tips that until now you thought were true and often took at face value. However, having reached the end of this book, I am going to broach a few essential points that, I believe, add to the quality of the book and set it apart.

FIRST—AND TO MY MIND MOST ESSENTIAL—WHAT is it that makes this book different? Without doubt, the most important characteristic of this book and its contents is its respect for the readers' intelligence, which underpins the book from its first to its last page.

Perhaps, because of my status as a cancer specialist and university professor, I could have gone for the easy option of thrusting dietary advice upon you from on high. I have never done this. Instead, I have tried to explain each time where the information came from, its degree of reliability, and how it fits in with all the scientific data on the matter.

I have explained to you the methods that allow researchers to reach a particular conclusion or hypothesis. To my mind, what is important is that by doing so, I have conveyed to you an understanding of the uncertainties that reign on our subject.

Once again, remember what I told you. Most of the studies that people use as a basis to claim that one thing is good for our health or that something else is bad are what we call "case-control" studies. We have seen the limits of these types of studies: how the subjects of the case and control groups struggle to recall what they were eating ten or fifteen years prior; how the questionnaires and the replies given to them are often inaccurate. But also and most importantly, it is impossible to guarantee that the case subjects are similar, let alone identical, to the control subjects, or even that the potential differences will be properly and comprehensively offset by the fact that ten or twenty times more control subjects will be used than case ones.

Thus, you have come to realize that when the "average" is arrived at, the study it is based on is imprecise and riddled with the risk of error.

When a paper states that a specific product increases or decreases our risk by 1%, 2%, or 3%, you are not being treated with serious respect.

I repeat myself once more: small differences found by such doubtful methods don't mean much.

When you are told so many portions per week of a particular food are toxic, but are not told the amount contained in a portion and whether it is similar to the portions eaten by the individuals participating in the study, as we saw with the red-meat example, once again you are not being taken seriously. When you are not told about the recent discovery of a new factor responsible for a particular cancer, a factor that was never taken into account in all the studies our experts were using to heap more restrictions on us, and that now makes these studies quite worthless, as happened with the human papillomavirus and mouth cancers, your legitimate right to know before making decision about your health and your life is not being respected. When a Finnish study concludes that eating a particular product is healthy for the Finns, and then there is an attempt to persuade the Japanese to do exactly the same, despite the fact that everything, absolutely everything, is different about the way in which these two nations go about eating and living in general, not to mention their major genetic differences, it just makes you want to laugh.

Finally, when the quacks, charlatans, or gurus—people who give medical advice but have no research to prove it—tell you that you ought to take a specific dietary supplement, they are playing the sorcerer's apprentice with you. However, don't forget that at the end of the day, unfortunately, you are the one likely to pay the price—you, who were naive enough to believe them without further reflection, without having the possibility of analyzing the evidence for yourself, and who blindly followed their fine words. Thus, by following a trend or through naïveté, thousands of you took vitamin A or beta-carotene, and more recently vitamin E, thinking that doing so would protect you from cancer.

You have also read in this book about all the studies of nutritional dietary supplements that had to be quickly stopped before they had even come to an end because it became clear that, far from doing good, these products were actually highly carcinogenic for humans, causing an increase in the number of cancers in the unfortunate volunteers who had been enlisted to take part in the studies.

My first message, then, at the end of this book is: Be critical. Do not simply believe anything and everything without an attempt to understand it.

Throughout this book, I have never stated anything using the authority of a present-tense verb that is not unquestionably an actual fact. For everything else, and you can check this, when I have given you information or advice concerning your diet, I have used words that indicate whether some food may be helpful.

No doubt, this is a habit acquired from carrying out research for over thirty years—a habit acquired by someone who has seen the nature of "scientific truth" change many times over the years.

How many times, for example, has it been announced that a remedy to cure cancer has been found, and how many times have we then had to grieve over the death of someone beloved by us who was nonetheless snatched away by this very disease?

Researchers are well aware that when handling results from any scientific research, our world and our lives are in reality far too complex not to carry on, in all modesty, using the conditional tense of a verb.

MY SECOND MESSAGE IS JUST AS IMPORTANT: Do not forget your common sense. Common sense, in the end, has always managed to guide humanity throughout its history. Common sense, yours as well as mine, must always subject new information on what to eat to critical analysis and scrutiny.

To some extent, what I am saying is, ask yourself questions whenever a claim is made that does not totally match up to reality as you see it. Give it some thought and try to understand why. Read over the information again; see where it comes from. Do not accept it as sacrosanct, and do not just go along with it with your eyes closed. It is grounded in this common sense that I would now like to address the following point. At the risk of disappointing you, I have to remind you here about what I have often mentioned in this book.

Men have an almost 50% "chance" of getting a cancer in their lifetime, and women have around a 30% chance. This means that cancer is a major risk, and as you now know, in the past four to five years it has become the leading cause of mortality in developed countries.

Confronted with a risk of such magnitude, you really need to understand this point (common sense also comes into play here): it is absolutely impossible to state that if you eat certain foods, you will not get cancer, or conversely, if you do eat them, you are certain to get a cancer (poor you!)! Never!

With everything I have explained here, it is likely that following our advice will lessen your intrinsic risk of cancer a little. Reduce it a little, but not put you out of harm's reach. Your dietary habits will increase or decrease your likelihood of getting a cancer or, if you have had one, of having a recurrence. But altering or adapting the way you eat cannot radically change your destiny.

Let's understand exactly what I am saying here. You are simply being warned about the extent, the scale, and the quantitative importance your nutrition can have on your current risk of developing a cancer. If this holds true for us, adults, we should be aware that when it comes to our children, this risk can be influenced to a far, far greater extent. Why? First, because everything that has a carcinogenic effect, including tobacco and food, has a far greater impact when acting on cells that are still relatively immature, and therefore fragile, as are children's cells. Next, because it very often takes ten to fifteen years and sometimes longer for a cancer to develop. This is, in a number of cases, the time that will have elapsed between the day when one cell in your body—one cell among a million billion—will become cancerous and the day when, the cell having silently multiplied in your body, it appears as a tumor, a cancer.

Remember how I told you that a tumor, a "lump," one centimeter (just over one-third of an inch) in diameter already contains a billion cancerous cells that cluster and stick together. If you then work out the calculation, knowing that with each cell division, one malignant cell will produce two daughter cells, and supposing that all the new cells are viable and capable in turn of dividing into two, more than thirty-three cell divisions are needed to go from one cancerous cell to a billion. If you calculate that one cell in, for example, a woman's mammary gland or a man's prostate requires on average three to four months to produce two cells, as this is the time it takes for this type of cell to create the genetic and cellular material needed to produce two identical daughter cells, you will see that it takes between ten and fifteen years to get from one cell to a tumor measuring one centimeter in diameter. In fact, it may take even longer, since lots of new cells that come into being with each division are unviable and die very quickly without producing any others. So this means there is even more time.

Indeed, a small cancer measuring one centimeter has a history that started a long time ago, a number of years before. That's the reason why we need to bear in mind that the 1.6 million or more patients who will be diagnosed with cancer annually in the United States over the next ten to fifteen years are already ill. They are already carrying in their bodies the beginnings of a cancer, a small tumor that is almost (or often even completely) invisible at this stage.

Screening is the only chance of diagnosing all these people's cancer very early on, when it may still be quite curable. When cancer has already been detected, it is too late for prevention. Therefore, for us adults, if we hope to lessen our risk of cancer, or, in the worst case scenario, to delay cancer's onset, by eating well and taking regular exercise we can only hope to do so to a measured extent, and not near 100%.

Those people who want to believe, as I have heard, that a particular diet is going to lower their risk of cancer or a cancer recurrence by over 50% are overly naive and gullible. It is not true; it cannot be true. They can undeniably lower their risk a little, but to think they can do so by over 50% is quite absurd.

MY THIRD MESSAGE IS RELATIVELY SIMPLE.

Ask yourself this question: How do we know that it is not dangerous for us to eat ceps and chanterelle mushrooms, but that we must never touch some others, such as deathcap mushrooms? In other words, how do we know, generally speaking, what is edible and what is not? It is actually relatively simple. Over the thousands of years since the first humanoid appeared on our good, old, planet Earth, man has tested everything, tasted everything, and tried everything over the generations in order to find something to eat.

How many of our ancestors would have eaten deathcap mushrooms, and also died from them, before their peers eventually worked out the connection between eating this mushroom and the subsequent death a day or two later? Some hundreds or thousands, I am sure. However, one day someone did make the connection, mentioned it to others, and warned them. From that moment on, deathcap mushrooms were not for eating, and nobody would ever touch them again, except by accident. What I am saying here about this mushroom that causes rapid death applies equally, of course, to all other foods that we now know we cannot eat safely.

However, you will ask, What does this story have to do cancer? The link is very simple, and even obvious. There is one thing you should tell yourself, and that is where my third message comes in. If a tribe, a people, a nation has developed particular eating habits throughout its history and over thousands of years, and has included particular products or recipes in its daily diet, and if this tribe, this people, this nation has nevertheless grown and survived through history and time, it is because its foods, its recipes, and its habits are not harmful. They do not result in any disease as fatal as cancer. This is very important, and we shall see why.

On several occasions we have talked about what the Japanese, the Chinese, the Finns, those from Crete, and the French and others eat. Throughout history, each of these peoples has developed eating habits to fit with its genetics (and also vice versa as a matter of fact), its environment, and terroir. Yet, all these customs, all these diets, are relatively different from each other. However, in spite of this, all these peoples have evolved and have succeeded in acquiring increasingly sophisticated technologies and knowledge that grow ever deeper and wider. They have reproduced themselves, they have managed to withstand time and the worst calamities, and they have become modern people. Not one of them has been decimated and wiped off the surface of the earth by cancer.

What I want to have you understand is that over the centuries these peoples could never have managed such a wonderfully well-adapted evolution if their eating habits had been systematically responsible for causing cancers. Conversely, none of these peoples, none of these nations, has remained untouched by cancer, and so this means that none of their eating habits has been capable of protecting them systematically from cancer either.

How do we look at these phenomena in relation to our study about the links between diet and cancer? We should simply tell ourselves that whatever their diet has consisted of over the centuries, it has been selected according to the terroir (that is, a particular environment able to produce certain foods). The diet could not really be carcinogenic because it was fitted to the surroundings and was bound to be varied, as was its preparation and cooking (to stay alive and develop demographically, each people had to use all available resources).

The very opposite is happening today, what I referred to earlier as the "Westernization" of our eating habits. It is no longer our history that tells us what to eat, or at least that is less and less common. Instead, advertising and the food-processing industry tell us. This trend toward "Westernization" makes us forget our terroirs and their recipes and products, encouraging us instead to all eat the same thing: processed products with added value for an industry that is forever dreaming up and producing these things. We are tending to eat a less diverse diet. Modern life is making us prepare our food in the same way, as we have seen: too rich, too much fat, and often toxic. We eat the same thing and do so too often. Look at the United States, a country without any specific long-standing gastronomic or culinary history, without the concept of terroir. It foreshadows what is likely to befall the rest of the West: pizza, beer, sugary soda, and television. Fast food with too much fat. Packets of potato chips full of acrylamide. Mega portions of meat that are too fatty and too highly grilled. And every age group eating too many dairy products.

These "neodiets" have not evolved out of a history that adapted a people to its terroir, so that each mother passed countless recipes on to her daughters over the generations, which ensured that a people developed harmoniously.

Our wealth lies here, in eating a diverse diet that is a result of our history—a diet that over the centuries has been proved to be harmless (even if this is bound to be relative, of course) and, what is more, has proved that it can take all these peoples respectful of their history and their environment into the future. I am telling you quite plainly that as long as you don't indulge every day, eating the occasional beef stew, drinking an odd glass of wine, or enjoying a nice piece of cheese is not carcinogenic. I am telling you this categorically—provided, of course, that you eat a varied, balanced diet that fits you and your lifestyle.

FINALLY, MY LAST MESSAGE is that of a man who has probably reached the culmination of his career, and even beyond that, of his life. It touches on the wonder I experience on a daily basis as I see all that we humans have conquered and all that we have dared to achieve. We have traveled into space and to the depths of the oceans; we have harnessed the energy in atoms and discovered the most extraordinary cures for most of the major diseases we have had to fight. We have reflected on life and wisdom; we have loved and produced offspring. We have created the most incredible arts and technological tools.

Over the centuries we humans have existed, we have done all this by venturing out from the dark corners of the cave where we were born, without light or fire, without any language, and terrorized by the world that surrounded us. We did all this because we were inherently and intrinsically driven by an unquenchable thirst for knowledge and progress. Because we felt intuitively that to master our environment, we had to be able to understand it, which gave rise to our permanent quest for knowledge and to our permanent risk-taking. If we had remained in the shelter of a cave, we would no doubt have avoided putting ourselves and our families at the risk of wild beasts or natural cataclysms, but there is no doubt either that our species would never have experienced the amazing destiny it has enjoyed—that we have enjoyed.

In a similar sort of way, I don't believe in an inward-looking society, fearful of everything, particularly when this touches on diet or daily life. We have made progress; progress enables us to be in better shape than our ancestors, and also to live far longer and be far healthier. To a large extent, subject to the provisos I have just pointed out, our diet has contributed greatly.

However, we are seeing emerge a kind of fear of progress. It is true that our lives are important and merit careful attention, but to preserve this life, at whatever cost, do we really want to turn our backs on progress? I don't go along with this attitude or posture that amounts to being afraid of everything and being willing to give up everything just so long as we can lead a nice, peaceful life.

AS A VERY YOUNG TEENAGER, I got up in the middle of the night on July 20, 1969, to watch Neil Armstrong on television, which was then black and white, land on the moon. I cried thinking about what had been my childhood dream, this marvelous dream that had just been made possible through man's intelligence and commitment to progress. And then I dreamed. For the rest of the night I dreamed about what this same progress would allow us to achieve in the future, and what I might have the opportunity of seeing one day during my lifetime. Progress then brought developments that never failed to amaze me, managing time and again to go far beyond my dreams. They made me proud to be a member of this seemingly quite unstoppable human race. Later on, much later on, having specialized in cancer, I cried again when, as a young intern in the Hôpital Saint-Louis in Paris, a small girl, six or seven years old, died in my arms from a devastating leukemia. Then again I dreamed that one day a cure would be discovered so that no more small children would ever die of leukemia. Nowadays, almost all of them are cured, thanks to advances in science. Their parents and their oncologists no longer shed tears either, or at any rate far less often. If we had been afraid of progress, if we had been frightened of trying, if the fear of making a mistake had made us helpless and stopped us in our tracks, then these dreams and many more besides would never have become a reality.

I am not one of those people who are frightened of progress. I do not believe that cell phones are carcinogenic. No study has ever proved this; quite the opposite, they all show that it is not true. I am not against research into GMOs. Nonetheless, I am most insistent that such research on both these topics be thoroughly regulated. Let us remind ourselves that humans can use the same scientific advance to promote life and progress or, conversely, as a weapon to spread death and suffering. Isn't radioactivity the prime example of this? It has given us radiotherapy that heals cancers, especially those cancers in very young children, yet at the same time it has led to a terrible nuclear arsenal that places humanity today at permanent risk. Should this discovery have been prevented? If this had happened, how many children would have been dead by now?

I dislike pesticides, weed killers, and all those horrible toxic things that are sprayed constantly over our earth. I would rather eat food that has been farmed using environmentally friendly methods. Yet I have to admit that there is no study to prove that doing so would lower my risk of cancer. That is the scientific truth.

I dislike reheating my food in a microwave oven because I find that it often comes out too soggy or overcooked. But microwave ovens do not give us cancer. That too is scientific truth.

How long would the list be if I were to set the record straight and convince you not to believe all the myths, so you didn't deprive yourself of pleasure because of misplaced fears?

Finally, at this time in my life, after thirty years of struggle—of desperate combat against cancer, my head full of all the faces I will never see again, all the voices I will never hear again—with a profound conviction, I tell myself that there are two things I cherish above all else and which are a source of great happiness for me.

First, life. Despite everything that can happen, I find life marvelous, and I battle on each day for it, because life is worth the battle. I feel this even more when I see one of my daughters smile, or when I take my wife's hand as we walk down the road together.

Then there is the future: the future I shall see and the one that I, unfortunately, will not get to see. However, if this future follows the course of the past, if it continues to be as full of discoveries, advances, and inspired inventions, this future is bound to be glorious for all those who live through it, from one generation to the next. Whether ultimately it is a glorious future will depend solely on them and what we will have passed on to them.

Appendix

···

AN ALPHABETICAL LIST OF FOODS
WITH ANTICANCER BENEFITS OR RISKS

Food	Healthy or harmful	Cancer ranking
Agar-agar (red seaweed)	A gelling agent that may aid digestion	Average
Agave syrup	Low antioxidant power; equivalent to sugar	Nothing to offer
Algae	Contain fucoxanthins and fucoidans with antioxidant properties	Very good
Almonds	Rich in vitamins	Good
Apple juice	Rich in antioxidant polyphenols and pectin	Average
Apples	Contain quercetin; high in fiber	Watch out for pesticides
Apricots	Rich in beta-carotene	Watch out for pesticides
Aromatic herbs	Rich in antioxidants	Good
Artichokes	Contain inulin, a prebiotic	Very good
Arugula	Contains flavonoids and in particular quercetin and carotenoids with antioxidant properties	Very good; eat plenty

(Table continues)

Food	Healthy or harmful	Cancer ranking
Aspartame	Tastes of sugar; zero calories	No problem
Avocado pears	Rich in polyunsaturated fatty acids and B-group vitamins	Very good
Bananas	Rich in prebiotic fiber	Very good
Barley	Rich in prebiotics	Very good
Basil	Contains aromatic polyphenols with anti-oxidant properties and anti-inflammatory ursolic acid	Very good
Battered, breaded fish	Check which fish is used (often lean); palm oil common	Not at all good
Beef	Try and get rid of the blood	No problem
Beets	A source of anthocyanins	Very good
Black olives	Rich in monounsaturated fatty acids; contain phenolic compounds	Good
Blackberries	A good source of anthocyanins	Very good
Black currants	Contain anthocyanins	Excellent
Blood sausage	High in heme iron	Not good
Blueberries	Contain tocotrienols and polyphenols with antioxidant properties	Very good; eat plenty
Bottled water	No pesticides, but some waters contain pollutants such as arsenic	Check before drinking
Brewers' yeast flakes	Rich in B-group vitamins (optimizing immunity)	Very good
Broccoli	Contains lots of folates glucoraphanin, isothiocyanates, and sulforaphane	Excellent
Brown butter sauce	Contains lots of lipidic peroxides	Not good
Brussels sprouts	Contains lots of indole compounds and isothiocyanates	Very good
Butter croissant	High in saturated fats	Average
Buttermilk	Rich in probiotics	Good
Candies	High in carbohydrates with no nutritional value	Not good
Canned vegetables	A source of vitamins, minerals (depending on the vegetable); check the salt content carefully	Very good, especially if tomatoes
Capers	Rich in quercetin	Excellent

Food	Healthy or harmful	Cancer ranking
Carrot juice	High in beta-carotene	Not good
Carrots	Rich in beta-carotene	Not too much
Cauliflower	Has almost no carotenoids; contains indole compounds	Very good
Celeriac (celery root)	Contains polyacetylenes that inhibit the growth of cancerous cells	Look out for pesticide residues
Cereals	A risk of aflatoxins	Average
Cheese	Rich in calcium and vitamin D	Very good for children; good for women (check the fat content); men over 50 should limit their intake
Cheese spread	High in saturated fatty acids and sodium	Not good
Cherries	A source of antioxidant anthocyanins and folates	Good
Chicken	Low in fat	Very good
Chicory	Rich in inulin; a prebiotic	Watch out for acrylamide
Chilis	A source of quercetin	Very good
Chinese cabbage	A source of indole compounds and isothiocyanates	Very good
Cinnamon	Anti-infective	Good
Coconut milk	High in fat (21%) and high in saturated fatty acids (18%)	Average
Cod, fresh	A lean fish; less contaminated than oily fish	Good
Cod-liver oil	Rich in omega-3	Good
Coffee	Anticarcinogenic properties seem due to it containing caffeine and polyphenols	Quite good
Condensed/evaporated milk	High in calcium, but watch out for the sugar	Not good
Coriander	Detoxifies heavy metals; contains aromatic polyphenols	Very good
Corn	A source of anthocyanins	Average
Crab	Often contaminated with heavy metals and PCBs	Exercise caution
Cranberries	A source of antioxidant anthocyanins	Very good

(Table continues)

Food	Healthy or harmful	Cancer ranking
Cream	High in saturated fats	Men over 50 should cut down
Dark chocolate	Contains antioxidants	Very good
Deli meats	High nitrate content (if industrially manufactured)	Exercise caution
Dill	A digestive stimulant	Very good
Doughnuts	High fat content with toxic compounds from the heated oil	Not good
Dried fruit	High sugar content	Average
Eggplant	Rich in insoluble fiber	Good
Eggs	Contains two carotenoids, lutein and zeaxanthin	Very good
Fennel	A low-calorie source of fiber and vitamin B9	Very good
Foie gras	Rich in iron	Good
French fries	High in fats and toxic compounds from the heated oil	Eat in moderation; use a good-quality oil
French toast	High acrylamide content	Not good
Fruit cordials	High in sugar	Not good
Fruit jelly/paste	High in sugar	Not good
Game	Fairly low in saturated fatty acids	Very good
Garden peas	A source of lutein	Good
Garlic	Contains sulfur compounds	Extraordinary
Ginger	When fresh, contains lots of vitamin C	Excellent
Gingerbread	High in sugar	Not very good
Glutamate	A flavor enhancer used in place of salt (3 times less sodium than standard table salt), but possible side effects: numbness in the neck, heart palpitations, etc.	Average
Goji berries	Contain *Lycium barbarum*, a polysaccharide with antioxidant properties	Good
Goose fat	High in saturated fatty acids	Good
Grape juice	Rich in flavonoids	Good
Grapefruit	A source of lycopene	Very good

Food	Healthy or harmful	Cancer ranking
Grapes	Contain numerous polyphenols, including resveratrol	Very good
Green olives	Less fat than black olives (12.5 g vs. 30 g) and rich in monounsaturated fatty acids; contain phenolic compounds	Very good
Grilled meats	High in polycyclic hydrocarbons	Not good
Guacamole	Due to avocado, high in polyunsaturated fatty acids and B-group vitamins; make your own as shop-bought guacamole is often very high in fat	Not bad
Guava	A source of lycopene	Good
Halibut	Often contaminated with heavy metals and PCBs	Exercise caution
Hard liquor	High concentration of ethanol; drink in moderation	Less than 30 g/day on average
Heavy cream	Contains lactobacillus; can be in fat	Average
Honey	Rich in fructose	Very good
Hummus	Rich in complex carbohydrates, but usually high in fat and calories too, so best to make your own	Not very good
Ice cream	High in fat, particularly saturated fats; high sugar content	Not good
Industrial-made croissant	Likely to contain trans fatty acids	Really not good
Jams	High in simple sugars without the goodness of fruit (vitamins, fiber, and minerals)	Watch out for the calories
Kefir	Lots of probiotics	Good
Ketchup	High in lycopene	Good
Kiwi	A source of lutein	Very good
Knackwurst	High in saturated fats, nitrites, and polyphosphates	Not very good
Lardons	High in salt and saturated fatty acids	Average
Lentils	A good source of plant proteins	Very good
Lettuce	A source of lutein	Good
Linseed	Rich in lignans (have to be crushed before they can be eaten)	Good

(Table continues)

Food	Healthy or harmful	Cancer ranking
Licorice	A digestive stimulant and a diuretic; raises blood pressure	Exercise caution
Lovage	Rich in flavonoids and quercetin in particular	Very good
Mangoes	Rich in beta-carotene	Good
Mayonnaise	Very high in fat	Not good
Melons	A source of lutein	Good
Milk	Contains lactose, calcium, and vitamin D	Very good for children; good for women; men over 50 should limit their intake
Mint	A good source of antioxidants; painkiller, antiseptic, and digestive stimulant	Very good
Muesli	High in fiber; however, do check carefully as some brands contain lots of sugar	Good
Mushrooms	A low-calorie food containing lots of useful vitamins	Very good
Mustard	Very acidic	Good
Nectarines	Contain bioflavonoids	Very good
Nutmeg	A digestive stimulant	Very good
Offal	Often high hemoglobin content	In moderation
Olive oil	Mainly made up of monounsaturated fatty acids	Very good
Orange juice	Contains fucoumarins, suspected of playing a role in the upsurge of malignant melanoma	If you spend time in the sun or are at risk of melanoma, exercise caution
Oranges	Rich in vitamin C and calcium	Good
Oysters	Rich in selenium	Good
Parsley	Rich in vitamin C and calcium	Very good
Parsnips	Contain apigenin, an antioxidant	Good
Peaches	Rich in beta-carotene	Watch out for pesticides
Peanut oil	Mainly made up of monounsaturated fatty acids	Good
Pears	Contain bioflavonoids	Watch out for pesticides

Food	Healthy or harmful	Cancer ranking
Peppers	Contain piperine, which makes turmeric more effective	Excellent
Pineapple juice	Contains bromelain, an enzyme that speeds up the digestion of fish and meat	Rather good
Pineapples	Contain bioflavonoids	Good
Plums	A good source of polyphenols	Good
Pollock	A lean fish, less contaminated than oily fish	Good
Pomegranate juice	Extremely rich in antioxidants, more than in green tea or wine	The best! Drink as much as you want!
Pomegranates	Contain ellagitannins, powerful antioxidants	Very good
Popcorn	Lots of complex carbohydrates and lipids; check how much salt and/or sugar is added; risk of acrylamide	Not at all good
Pork	The fat content varies according to which cut you use	Don't eat the fat
Potato chips	High acrylamide content	Exercise caution; very bad
Potatoes	Complex carbohydrates and vitamin C in the skin; antioxidant properties	Good
Pumpkins	Rich in carotenoids	Good
Quinoa, seeds	Very high in magnesium, non-heme iron; a source of plant proteins; high in fiber	Very good
Rabbit	A useful source of polyunsaturated fatty acids	Very good
Radishes, black winter	Contain sulfur compounds	Very good
Rapeseed oil	Contains polyunsaturated fatty acids; unstable if exposed to heat and light	Average
Raspberries	Rich in anthocyanins; high mineral density	Good
Red cabbage	Contains anthocyanins	Good
Red kidney beans	A source of anthocyanins	Good
Red onions	A source of anthocyanins	Excellent
Rice	High in complex carbohydrates	Very good

(Table continues)

Food	Healthy or harmful	Cancer ranking
Rutabaga	A source of indole compounds	Good
Saccharose	High in calories (400 kcal/100 g)	No problem
Salmon	Often contaminated with heavy metals and PCBs	Exercise caution
Salmon taramasalata	A high-energy, high-fat food; source of omega-3 (depending on which oil is used)	Average
Salt	Incriminated in some stomach cancers	In moderation
Sardines in sunflower oil	Poor omega-3 and omega-6 balance	Good
Savory aperitif snacks	High acrylamide content	Not good
Sea urchins	Rich in iodine	Very good
Semolina, couscous, durum wheat	A good source of proteins and complex carbohydrates; always try to eat whole wheat as the outer husk contains antioxidant compounds	Good
Sesame, seeds	High in protein and fiber	Very good
Shrimp	Low in fat and little contamination	Very good
Smoked fish	High in salt and polycyclic aromatic hydrocarbons	Not good
Smoothie	Rich in antioxidants but also in simple sugars	Average
Sodas	Lots of simple sugars	Not good
Sorbet	Often high in simple sugars; best to make your own sorbets using high antioxidant fruits	Average; don't overdo it
Soy	Contains phytoestrogens	Good
Soy sauce	Lots of salt	Not very good
Sparerib of pork	Fatty: 23.6% fats and the way it's cooked is carcinogenic	Not at all good
Spelt, seeds	High in fiber, plant proteins, and magnesium	Very good
Spinach	Rich in carotenoid and calcium	Good
Spreads	High in fat and sugar	Not very good
Star anise	A digestive stimulant with antiseptic action	Very good

Food	Healthy or harmful	Cancer ranking
Steak tartare	Raw meat; rich in heme iron	Good
Stevia	High sweetening power	Not yet known
Strawberries	Contain calcium and iron, as well as anthocyanins	Good
Sunchokes	Contain inulin, which has a prebiotic action	Good
Sunflower oil	Contains polyunsaturated fatty acids; unstable if exposed to heat and light	Good
Sushi	High in polyunsaturated fatty acids but also often contaminated	Exercise caution
Sweet peppers	Contain bioflavonoids	Very good
Sweet potatoes	Contain complex carbohydrates, and anthocyanins with antioxidant properties; rich in beta-carotene	Good
Tap water	Depending on your area, may contain nitrates, pesticides, and/or arsenic	Check before drinking
Tapenade (garlic and black olives)	High in monounsaturated fatty acids but often high in fat	Not very good
Tea	Contains epigallocatechin-3-gallate	Very good
Tofu	Contains phytoestrogens	Very good
Tomatoes	A source of lycopene	Excellent, especially for men
Tomatoes, dried in oil	Contain very bioavailable lycopene	Very good
Tuna	Often contaminated with heavy metals and PCBs	Exercise caution, especially with red tuna
Turmeric	A yellow pigment containing curcumin	Excellent
Turnips	Contain indole compounds and sulfur heterosides	Very good
Vanilla, extract	Antioxidant	Good
Vegetable stock	A good source of vitamins, minerals, and antioxidants	Very good
Verbena tea, herbal tea	Try and use different types of herbal tea; calms digestion	Very good
Vinegar	A digestive stimulant	No problem

(Table continues)

Food	Healthy or harmful	Cancer ranking
Walnuts	Contain omega-3	Very good
Watercress	A source of indole compounds	Very good
Watermelons	A source of lycopene	Very good
White bread	Contains little fiber	Good
White onion	Contains selenium with antioxidant properties	Excellent
Whole-wheat bread	High in fiber with lots of complex carbohydrates	Very good
Wine	Contains resveratrol, a powerful antioxidant with known anticancer properties	Very good, but drink in moderation
Yogurt	Contains living bacteria: probiotics	Good
Zucchini	Contain carotenoids	Very good

Glossary

adenocarcinoma — A malignant tumor in cells that make up the glands

aflatoxins — Toxins produced by certain molds when temperature and humidity conditions are high

apoptosis — One of the processes for cell death that take place in an organism and by which cells set in motion their own self-destruction in response to a signal

arsenic — A mineral element, toxic in almost all its forms

bacillus — An elongated bacteria

bacteria — A unicellular microorganism without a nucleus (prokaryote) that does not belong to either the animal or the vegetable kingdom; certain bacteria can be pathogenic

bioactive — A compound that interacts positively with the body

biocompounds — Compounds from the living world

biological half-life — The time required for the activity of a radioactive substance to be halved

butyrate or butyric acid — A chemical compound produced by the bacteria found in the digestive tract with beneficial properties for digestive health

cadmium — A mineral element, a heavy metal that when absorbed in food, accumulates in the liver and kidneys

carcinogen — Any element that is likely to induce the onset of a cancer

carcinogenic — Capable of causing the onset of cancer

cell	The fundamental element that all living creatures are made of
cell differentiation	The process by which cells become specialized to create a specific organ
chromosomes	Bodies found inside the nucleus of a cell that are made up of DNA and therefore provide genetic information
cytochrome	A respiratory pigment found in all living cells
detoxification	The mechanism that ensures that undesirable molecules (pesticides, medication) get eliminated along with the waste produced by cells as they function
dioxins	Substances found in the environment and in the food chain that are formed by natural and industrial combustion
DNA (deoxyribonucleic acid)	A vital component for the chromosomes in the cell's nucleus
enzyme	A substance capable of accelerating or bringing about certain chemical processes without being altered itself
estrogens	Hormones involved in female reproduction
fermentation	The transformation of certain organic substances from the action of enzymes produced by microorganisms
fertilization	The fusion between a sperm and an ovum that produces a single cell, the egg from which an embryo will form
fiber	A substance found in foodstuffs made from plants; helps move the digestion process along and makes us feel full
free radical	Atom or group of atoms produced because the human body uses oxygen; involved in numerous cell processes but may also be responsible for the onset of certain diseases linked with aging
gene	A sequence of nucleotides that provides genetic information to control the expression of a specific characteristic

genetic	Having to do with genes and heredity
genetic code	An "alphabet" that allows the organism to translate the genetic information the DNA is carrying
genistein	A compound present mostly in soy that works in a similar way to female hormones
genotoxic	A substance or radiation that may induce a mutation of the genome in particular
glucoraphanin	A molecule that belongs to the glucosinolates family, containing a sulfur atom; found chiefly in broccoli
glutathione S-transferase	An enzyme that activates the detoxification reaction in the liver
glycemic index	A criterion used to classify foods according to the extent to which they raise the blood sugar level after they have been ingested
growth factor	A natural substance capable of stimulating cell growth, proliferation, and differentiation
heavy metals	High-density metallic elements, including lead, cadmium, mercury, and arsenic
hemoglobin	A complex molecule made up of proteins and iron, particularly involved with transporting oxygen in blood; gives blood its red color
hereditary	Something that is passed on from parents to off-spring according to the laws of genetics
hydrogen peroxide	A chemical compound with powerful oxidizing properties that may be responsible for serious cell damage; usually called "oxygenated water"
hydroxyl radical	A compound formed during cell metabolism, and mostly responsible for the damage caused to the body by free radicals
immune system	A complex set of cells, organs, and molecules that enables the body to protect itself from infections and undesirable elements
indole	A blue pigment with antioxidant properties
isothiocyanates	Substances found in significant amounts in cru-

ciferous vegetables (cabbages, Brussels sprouts, broccoli)

lead
A mineral element naturally present in the environment and used in numerous industrial applications; chronic lead poisoning, called "saturnism," has long been recorded

lycopene
A carotenoid that gives tomatoes and other fruits their red color and acts as a powerful antioxidant

malnutrition
A pathological state caused by a deficiency or a surplus of one or more nutrients

metabolism
All the reactions that continually take place, enabling a living organism to function and survive

methylmercury
The form of organic mercury most commonly found in the environment; found in particular in fish and other marine products, due to bioaccumulation

mutation
A modification of the genetic information carried by DNA; may be of no significance or may disrupt the workings of the cell, leading at times to cancer

nutrients
All the components we get from what we eat and drink and that we need for our bodies to grow and function properly; derived from digesting food and can be directly used by cells

nutrigenomics
A science that studies how genes interact with what we eat and drink

omega-3
A family of polyunsaturated fatty acids found chiefly in oily fish, linseed, walnuts, and rapeseed; defined as essential fatty acids, as the body needs them to function properly but it cannot produce them itself

oncogene
A gene that encourages or causes the onset of tumors

oxidative stress
An oxidation process caused by free radicals in the cell components

p53
A protein involved in protecting the body from DNA lesions

parabens
Preservatives

peroxidase	An enzyme that activates oxidation reactions
persistent organic pollutants (POPs)	Chemical substances that remain in the environment and accumulate in the tissues of living organisms; potentially harmful to health
photosynthesis	A process that enables plants to transform the energy from light into energy their cells can use
phytocompounds	Substances that are found only in plants
piperine	A compound found in pepper that gives it its spicy taste
polychlorinated biphenyls (PCBs)	Chlorinated chemical derivatives that decompose naturally very slowly so they remain in the environment and are hardly soluble in water
polycyclic aromatic hydrocarbons (PAHs)	Harmful chemical compounds that are formed during some cooking processes
polyp	A soft, benign tumor
polysaccharides	Carbohydrates made of long chains, such as starch, cellulose, and glycogen
prebiotics	Fibers that are indigestible by humans so they are used and transformed by the bacteria in the intestines; stimulate the growth of certain healthy bacteria
probiotics	Living microorganisms found in some foodstuffs; health-giving to those who eat them
protein	A molecule that is indispensable for the structure and function of a cell and organism
Pyralene	The commercial name for a PCB-based product
radon	An inert, radioactive, natural gas; odorless, colorless, and tasteless
retinoic acid	One of the forms of vitamin A that helps the eyes function properly and the skin grow
scavenger	Used to describe a meal that is eaten to lessen or eliminate the negative effects of a foodstuff
selenium	A trace element with powerful antioxidant activity;

	necessary for certain detoxifying enzymes to function correctly
senescence	Or aging: all the alterations that time brings about in human beings
steroid hormones	Hormones synthesized in the body from cholesterol
sulforaphane	A phytonutrient (a nutrient of plant origin, different from vitamins and minerals), one of its properties being to lower the risk of cancer; broccoli contains a lot of sulforaphane
sweetener	A substance that tastes sweet but contains fewer calories than sugar
symbiotic	A combination of probiotics and prebiotics that stimulates the appearance of beneficial bacteria in the digestive system
testosterone	A hormone that acts on the development of genital organs and male secondary sexual characteristics
toxin	A toxic substance created by a living organism that can result in harmful effects for health
trace elements	Mineral elements that the body needs in very small quantities to function properly
tumor	Excrescence of a tissue that may be benign or malignant
virus	A very tiny infectious agent that uses the components in a host cell to multiply
vitamin	An organic substance, tiny amounts of which are vital for the body to grow and function properly, but which the body cannot synthesize
vitamin D	A vital vitamin for the absorption of calcium for bones; also helps with the absorption of phosphorus

List of Abbreviations

AFSSA (now ANSES)	French Food Safety Agency (Agence française de securité sanitaire des aliments)
AIDS	acquired immunodeficiency syndrome
ASEF	French Association of Environmental Health (Association Santé Environnement France)
BMI	body mass index
CAMI	French Association of Cancer, Martial Arts and Information (Cancer Arts Martiaux et Information: www.sportetcancer.com)
CD	compact disc
DGCCRF	French Directorate General for Competition, Consumer Affairs and Repression of Fraud (Direction Générale de la Concurrence, de la Consommation et de la Repression des Fraudes)
DNA	deoxyribonucleic acid
DRASS	French Regional Directorate of Health and Social Affairs (Direction Régionale des Affaires Sanitaires et Sociales)
EGCG	epigallocatechin-3-gallate
ENT	ear, nose, and throat (otorhinolaryngology)
HAT	histone acetyltransferase
HDAC	histone deacetylase
HPV	human papillomavirus
HRT	hormone replacement therapy

IARC	International Agency for Research on Cancer
IGF1	insulin-like growth factor
INCA	French National Cancer Institute (Institut National du Cancer)
INVS	French Institute for Public Health Surveillance (Institut National de Veille Sanitaire)
MUFAs	monounsaturated fatty acids
NHS	National Health Service
PCB	polychlorinated biphenyls
PNNS	French Nutrition and Health Program (Programme national nutrition santé)
POP	persistent organic pollutant
PSA	prostate-specific antigen
PUFAs	polyunsaturated fatty acids
SFAs	saturated fatty acids
TFAs	trans fatty acids
WCRF	World Cancer Research Fund
WHO	World Health Organization

A Note on References

....

Note: For every piece of important information contained in this book, we have indicated where it was taken from in the scientific bibliographical references.

The original documents we used to write this book can be easily found by anyone.

We have made frequent reference to the report that the World Research Cancer Fund (WCRF) published in 2007: *Food, Nutrition, Physical Activity, and the Prevention of Cancer: A Global Perspective.* We mentioned the (rare) occasions where we have disagreed with the report.

The information supplied by the French Food Safety Agency has been of great help to us. This organization does wonderful work to ensure the quality of the food we eat, as do other French bodies: French Directorate General for Competition, Consumer Affairs and Repression of Fraud; French General Directorate of Health; French Regional Directorate of Health and Social Affairs; and French Institute for Public Health Surveillance. Their websites are often of great interest and full of relevant information.

Lastly, to keep things clear, we have rounded off most of the numbers given, to avoid weighing them down with decimal points.

Notes

....

Chapter 1: Cancer: Choosing Prevention

1. Curado M. P., Edwards B., Shin H. R., Storm H., Ferlay M., Boyle P. (eds.), *Cancer Incidence in Five Continents*, vol. 9, IARC Scientific Publication, no. 160 (Lyon, International Agency for Research on Cancer, 2007).

2. Ibid.

3. Ibid. Centers for Disease Control and Prevention, *Fast Stats: AIDS and HIV*, mortality data, 2009, available at http://www.cdc.gov/nchs/fastats/aids-hiv.htm (accessed November 14, 2012).

4. American Cancer Society, *Cancer Facts and Figures 2014*, "Estimated New Cancer Cases and Deaths by Sex for All Sites, US, 2014," available at www .cancer.org/acs/groups/content/@research/documents/webcontent/acspc-04215 .pdf (accessed October 6, 2014).

5. American Cancer Society, *Cancer Facts and Figures, 2014*.

6. Centers for Disease Control and Prevention, *National Vital Statistics System: Mortality Tables*, Cause of death (based on the tenth revision, International Classification of Diseases, second edition, 2004), race, sex, and age, 2009, available at http://www.cdc.gov/nchs/nvss/mortality_tables.htm (accessed November 14, 2012).

7. Centers for Disease Control and Prevention, *Smoking—Attributable Mortality, Years of Potential Life Lost, and Productivity Losses—United States, 2000–2004*, table, available at http//www.cdc.gov/mmwr/preview/mmwrhtml/mm5745a3 .htm tab (accessed November 14, 2012).

8. American Cancer Society, *Cancer Facts and Figures 2014*, available at www.cancer
.org/acs/groups/content/@epidemiology/surveillance/documents/document/
acspc-026238.pdf (accessed July 28, 2014), p. 4.

9. Curado M. P., et al. (eds.), *Cancer Incidence in Five Continents*.

10. Preetha Anand, "Cancer Is a Preventable Disease that Requires Major Lifestyle
Changes," *Pharm. Res.*, September 2008, 25 (9), pp. 2097–2116.

11. Académie des Sciences, *Les causes du cancer en France* [The Causes of cancer in France], available at http://www.academie-sciences.fr/activite/rapport
/rapport130907.pdf (accessed April 16, 2014).

12. Each year tobacco kills 443,000 people prematurely in the United States.
Centers for Disease Control and Prevention, *Smoking & Tobacco Use*: *Tobacco-
Related Mortality*, available at http://www.cdc.gov/tobacco/data_statistics
/fact_sheets/health_effects/tobacco_related_mortality/ (accessed November
14, 2012).

13. National Cancer Institute Fact Sheet, "'Light' Cigarettes and Cancer Risk,"
October 28, 2010, www.cancer.gov/cancertopics/factsheet/Tobacco/light
-cigarettes (accessed August 14, 2014).

14. Khayat D., *Les Chemins de l'espoir* [The Paths of Hope] (Paris, Odile Jacob,
2003).

15. Milner J. A., "Nutrition and cancer: Essential elements for a roadmap," *Cancer
Lett.*, 2008, 269, pp. 189–198.

16. Jauzein F., Cros N., *Différents types d'études épidémiologiques* [Different types
of epidemiological studies], 2005, available at: http://acces.ens-lyon.fr/acces
/ressources/sante/epidemiologie/niveau_preuve/types_etudes_epidem (accessed
April 16, 2014).

17. Milner J. A., "Nutrition and cancer."

Chapter 2: What Is Cancer?

1. World Cancer Research Fund, *Food, Nutrition, Physical Activity, and the Prevention of Cancer: A Global Perspective* (Washington, D.C., American Institute
for Cancer Research, 2007).

2. Ibid.

3. Lampe J. W., "Diet genetic polymorphism, detoxification, and health risk," *Altern. Ther. Health Med.*, 2007, 13, pp. S108–S111.

4. World Cancer Research Fund, *Food, Nutrition, Physical Activity, and the Prevention of Cancer.*

5. Ibid.

Chapter 3: Is Fish a Health Food or a Health Risk?

1. Liperoti R., Landi F., Fusco O., Bernabei R., Onder G., "Omega-3 polyunsaturated fatty acids and depression: A review of the evidence," *Curr. Pharm. Des.*, 2009, 15 (36), pp. 4165–4172.

2. ANSES [French Food Safety Agency], *Gras ou pas gras mon poisson?* [Is my fish oily or not?], 2009, available at http://www.anses.fr/Documents/AFSSA -Fi-Poisson-F5.pdf (accessed March 29, 2010).

3. ACCES, *Quels poisons consommer?* [Which fish should we eat?], 2008. (Consumption File of *Défi pour la Terre*, pp. 1–5, available at http://www.acces .lautre.net (accessed July 26, 2014).

4. World Cancer Research Fund, *Food, Nutrition, Physical Activity, and the Prevention of Cancer.*

5. US Food and Drug Administration, "Foodborne Illness and Contaminants," www.fda.gov/Food/FoodborneIllnessContaminants/default.htm (accessed October 6, 2014).

6. World Health Organization, International Program on Chemical Safety (WHO-IPCS), *Environmental Health Criteria 101, Methylmercury* (Geneva, International Program on Chemical Safety, 1990), available at http://www .inchem.org/documents/ehc/ehc/ehc101.htm (accessed March 8, 2010).

7. Direction générale de la santé [French General Directorate of Health], *Étude sur la teneur en métaux dans l'alimentation* [Study on metal content in foods], (Paris, La Diagonale des métaux, 1992).

8. International Agency for Research on Cancer (IARC), *Monographs on the Evaluation of Carcinogenic Risks to Humans*, available at http://monographs.iarc .fr/ENG/Classification/index.php (accessed March 7, 2010).

9. IARC, *Évaluation globale de la cancérogénicité pour l'homme, 2009* [Mono-

graphs on the evaluation of carcinogenic risks to humans], available at http://monographs.iarc.fr/FR/Classification/crthall.php (accessed March 29, 2010).

10. International Agency for Research on Cancer (IARC), *Monographs on the Evaluation of Carcinogenic Risks to Humans*, available at http://monographs.iarc.fr/ENG/Classification/index.php (accessed March 7, 2010).

11. World Health Organization (WHO), *Dioxins and Their Effects on Human Health*, 2007, available at http://www.who.int/mediacentre/factsheets/fs225/en/index.html (accessed March 8, 2010).

12. Kaushik S., "Les dioxines et les PCB chez le poisson" [Dioxins and PCBs in fish], *Dossier de l'environnement de l'INRA*, no. 26, pp. 102–107, available at http://www.inra.fr/dpenv/pdf/kaush2d26.pdf (accessed July 27, 2014).

13. World Health Organization (WHO), *Dioxins and Their Effects on Human Health.*

14. European Food Safety Authority (EFSA), "Opinion of the Scientific Panel on Contaminants in the Food Chain (CONTAM) related to the safety assessment of wild and farmed fish," *EFSA Journal*, July 11, 2006, available at http://www.efsa.europa.eu/EFSA/efsa_locale-1178620753816_1178620762697.htm (accessed April 16, 2014).

15. AFSSA [French Food Safety Agency], *Avis de l'Agence Française de sécurité sanitaire des aliments relatif à l'établissement de teneurs maximales pertinentes en polychlorobiphényles que ne sont pas de type dioxine (PCB "non dioxin-like," PCB-NDL) dans divers aliments*, 2007 [Advice from the French Food Safety Agency about establishing relevant maximum polychlorobiphenyl contents that are non dioxin-like PCB-NDL in various foods, 2007], referral no. 2006-SA-0305.

16. Ribeira D., Loock T., Soler P., Narbonne J.-F., "Mise en évidence d'effets à long terme lors d'expositions courtes (accidentelles). Perspectives méthodologiques pour les evaluations des risques" [Highlighting long-term effects from short (accidental) exposures. Methodological perspectives for risk assessments], *Étude Record*, 2006–2007, no. 06-0665/1A.

17. IARC, *Monographs on the Evaluation of Carcinogenic Risks to Humans.*

18. Davis J. A., Hetzel F., Oram J. J., McKee L. J., "Polychlorinated biphenyls (PCBs) in San Francisco Bay," *Environ. Res.* 2007, 105(1), pp. 67–86.

19. Oken E., Choi A. L., Karagas M. R., Mariën K., Rheinberger C. M., Schoeny R., Sunderland E., Korrick S., "Which Fish Should I Eat? Perspectives Influencing Fish Consumption Choices," *Env. Health Persp.*, 2012, 120.6, pp. 790–798.

20. Howsam M., Grimalt J. O., Guinó E., Navarro M., Martí-Ragué J., Peinado M. A., Capellá G., Moreno V., "Organochlorine exposure and colorectal cancer risk," *Environ. Health Perspect.*, 2004, 112 (15), pp. 1460–1466.

21. Hordell L., Calberg M., Hardell K., Bjornfoth H., Wickbom G., Ionescu M., "Decreased survival in pancreatic cancer patients with high concentrations of organochlorines in adipose tissue," *Biomed. Pharmacother.*, 2007, 61 (10), pp. 659–664.

22. ASEF [French Association of Environmental Health]–WWF, *Imprégnation aux PCB des riverains du Rhône* [PCB impregnation with Rhône riverside dwellers], May 2008, available at: http://www.asef-asso.fr/mon-alimentation/notre -etude-pch/10-mai-2008-notre-etude-sur-les-pcb (accessed March 8, 2010).

23. Leblanc J.-C. (ed.), *Étude Calipso.*

24. Ibid.

25. AFSSA, "Consommation de poisson et méthylmercure [Consumption of fish and methylmercury], press release July 25, 2006, available at http://www.afssa .fr/Documents/PRES2006CP013.pdf (accessed March 8, 2010).

26. U.S. Food and Drug Administration and U.S. Environmental Protection Agency, "What You Need to Know about Mercury in Fish and Shellfish, 2004 EPA and FDA Advice for Women Who Might Become Pregnant, Women Who are Pregnant, Nursing Mothers, Young Children," publication EPA-823-F-04-009, available at www.fda.gov/downloads/Food/Foodborneillness Contaminants/UCM182158.pdf (accessed May 9,2014).

27. Hites R. A., Foran J. A., Carpenter D. O., Hamilton C. M., Knuth B. A., Schwager S. J., "Global assessment of organic contaminants in farmed salmon," *Science*, 2004, 303 (5655), pp. 226–229.

28. AFSSA, AFSSA press release following the publication of the survey *L'Analyse globale des contaminants chimiques dans le saumon d'élevage* [Global analysis of chemical contaminants in farmed salmon], January 9, 2004, available at http://w3.rennes.inra.fr/inraquac/actualites/afssa-dioxine (accessed April 16, 2014).

29. WHO, *PCBs and Dioxins in Salmon: Organochlorine Contamination of Salmon,*" January 20, 2004, available at http://www.who.int/foodsafety/chem/pcbsa lmon/en/print.html (accessed March 8, 2010).

30. EFSA, "Opinion of the Scientific Panel on Contaminants in the Food Chain (CONTAM)."

31. Kaushik S., "Les dioxines et les PCB chez le poisson."

32. AFSSA, "Le poisson sous haute surveillance" [Fish under high surveillance], available at www.afssa.fr/Documents/APR-mg-aPropos23.pdf (accessed July 27, 2014).

33. Leblanc J.-C. (ed.), *Étude Calipso.*

Chapter 4: Red Meat

1. U.S. Census Bureau, *Statistical Abstract of the United States*, "Table 217. Per Capita Consumption of Major Food Commodities: 1980 to 2009," available at www.census.gov/compendia/statab/2012/tables/12s0217.pdf (accessed May 9, 2014).

2. World Cancer Research Fund, *Food, Nutrition, Physical Activity, and the Prevention of Cancer: A Global Perspective* (Washington, D.C., American Institute for Cancer Research, 2007).

3. Ibid.

4. Ibid.

5. Willett W. C., Stampfer M. J., Colditz G. A., Rosner B. A., Speizer F. E., "Relation of meat, fat, and fiber intake to the risk of colon cancer in a prospective study among women," *N. Engl. J. Med.*, 1990, 323 (24), pp. 1664–1672.

6. Wei E. K., Giovannucci E., Wu K., Rosner B., Fuchs C. S., Willett W. C., Colditz G. A., "Comparison of risk factors for colon and rectal cancer," *Int. J. Cancer*, 2004, 108 (3), pp. 433–442.

7. Ibid.

8. Goldbohm R. A., Van den Brandt P. A., Van't Veer P., Brants H. A., Dorant E., Sturmans F., Hermus R. J., "A prospective cohort study on the relation between meat consumption and the risk of colon cancer," *Cancer Res.*, 1994, 54 (3), pp. 718–723.

9. Knekt P., Steineck G., Järvinen R., Hakulinen T., Aromaa A., "Intake of fried meat and risk of cancer: A follow-up study in Finland," *Int. J. Cancer*, 1994, 59 (6), pp. 756–760.

10. Gaard M., Tretli S., Løken E. B., "Dietary factors and risk of colon cancer: A prospective study of 50,535 young Norwegian men and women," *Eur. J. Cancer Prev.*, 1996, 5 (6), pp. 445–454.

11. Norat T., Bingham S., Ferrari P., Slimani N., Jenab M., Mazuir M., Overvad K., Olsen A., Tjønneland A., Clavel F., Boutron-Ruault M. C., Kesse E., Boeing H., Bergmann M. M., Nieters A., Linseisen J., Trichopoulou A., Trichopoulos D., Tountas Y., Berrino F., Palli D., Panico S., Tumino R., Vineis P., Bueno-de-Mesquita H. B., Peeters P. H., Engeset D., Lund E., Skeie G., Ardanaz E., González C., Navarro C., Quirós J. R., Sanchez M. J., Berglund G., Mattisson I., Hallmans G., Palmqvist R., Day N. E., Khaw K. T., Key T. J., San Joaquin M., Hémon B., Saracci R., Kaaks R., Riboli E., "Meat, fish, and colorectal cancer risk: The European Prospective Investigation into Cancer and Nutrition," *J. Natl. Cancer Inst.*, 2005, 97 (12), pp. 906–916. See p. 911.

12. Truswell A. S., "Meat consumption and cancer of the large bowel," *Eur. J. Clin. Nutr.*, 2002, 56, suppl. 1, pp. S19–S24.

13. Ibid.

14. Gaard M., et al., "Dietary factors and risk of colon cancer."

15. AFSSA [French Food Safety Agency], *French Food Composition Table: Table CIQUAL 2012*, available at: http://pro.anses.fr/TableCIQUAL/ (accessed February 20, 2014).

16. U.S. Department of Agriculture (USDA), Agricultural Research Service, *National Nutrient Database for Standard Reference*, available at http://www.nal.usda.gov/fnic/foodcomp/search/ (accessed March 20, 2010).

17. AFSSA, *Table CIQUAL 2012*.

18. USDA, *National Nutrient Database for Standard Reference*.

19. CIV [Center for Meat Information], *Niveau de consummation de viande en France* [Level of meat consumption in France], available at http://www.civ-viande.org/4-139-nutrition-niveau-de-consommation-de-viande-en-france.html (accessed March 20, 2010).

20. U.S. Census Bureau, *Statistical Abstract of the United States*, "Table 217. Per Capita Consumption of Major Food Commodities: 1980 to 2009."

21. AFSSA, *Table CIQUAL 2012*.

22. USDA, *National Nutrient Database for Standard Reference*.

23. AFSSA, *Étude individuelle nationale des consommations alimentaires 2* [Individual National Study of Food Consumption 2] *(INCA 2) 2006–2007*, 2009, available at www.anses.fr/Documents/PASER-Ra-INCA2.pdf (accessed December 11, 2014).

24. USDA, *USDA Economic Research Service*, available at http://www.ers.usda.gov /topics/animalproducts.aspx#.VBbtlS5_vE1

25. U.S. Census Bureau, *Statistical Abstract of the United States*, "Table 217. Per Capita Consumption of Major Food Commodities: 1980 to 2009."

26. CIV, *Niveau de consummation de viande en France*.

27. Cross A. J., Pollock J. R. A., Bingham S. A., "Haem, not protein or inorganic iron, is responsible for endogenous intestinal N-nitrosation arising from red meat 7," *Cancer Res.*, 2003, 63, pp. 2358–2360.

28. Nelson R. L., "Iron and colorectal cancer risk: Human studies," *Nutr. Rev.*, 2001, 59 (5), pp. 140–148.

29. Vano Y.-A., Rodrigues M.-J., Schneider S.-M., "Lien épidémiologique entre comportement alimentaire et cancer: exemple du cancer colorectal" [Epidemiological link between eating habits and cancer: colorectal cancer as an example], *Bulletin du cancer*, 2009, 96 (6), pp. 647–658.

30. Lipkin M., "Biomarkers of increased susceptibility to gastrointestinal cancer: New application to studies of cancer prevention in human subjects," *Cancer Res.*, 1988, 48 (2), pp. 235–245.

31. Sesink A. L., Termont D. S., Kleibeuker J. H., Van der Meer R., "Red meat and colon cancer: The cytotoxic and hyperproliferative effects of dietary heme," *Cancer Res.*, 1999, 59 (22), pp. 5704–5709.

32. Sesink A. L., Termont D. S., Kleibeuker J. H. Van der Meer R., "Red meat and colon cancer: Dietary haem-induced colonic cytotoxicity and epithelial hyperproliferation are inhibited by calcium," *Carcinogenesis*, 2001, 22 (10), pp. 1653–1659.

33. Ibid.

Chapter 5: Do Dairy Products and Eggs Help Prevent Cancer?

1. Wollowski I., Rechkemmer G., Pool-Zobel B. L., "Protective role of probiotics and prebiotics in colon cancer," *Am. J. Clin. Nutr.*, 2001, 73 (2), suppl., pp. 451S–455S.

2. Lomer M. C., Parkes G. C., Sanderson J. D., "Review article: Lactose intolerance in clinical practice—myths and realities," *Aliment. Pharmacol. Ther.*, 2008, 27, pp. 93–103.

3. Liong M. T., "Roles of probiotics and prebiotics in colon cancer prevention: Postulated mechanisms and *in vivo* evidence," *Int. J. Mol. Sci.*, 2008, 9 (5), pp. 854–863.

4. Ibid.

5. Wollowski I., et al., "Protective role of probiotics and prebiotics in colon cancer."

6. Ibid.

7. Ibid.

8. Lomer M. C., et al., "Review article."

9. Ibid.

10. *Diet for Lactose Intolerance: Lactose Content of Dairy Foods*, Gastro Net, http://www.gastro.net.au/diets/lactose.html (accessed July 27, 2014).

11. Ibid.

12. Swagerty D. L. Jr., Walling A. D., Klein R. M., "Lactose intolerance," *Am. Fam. Physician*, 2002, 65 (9), pp. 1845–1850.

13. Torniainen S., Hedelin M., Autio V., Rasinperä H., Bälter K. A., Klint A., Bellocco R., Wiklund F., Stattin P., Ikonen T., Tammela T. L., Schleutker J., Grönberg H., Järvelä I., "Lactase persistence, dietary intake of milk, and the risk for prostate cancer in Sweden and Finland," *Cancer Epidemiol. Biomarkers Prev.*, 2007, 16 (5), pp. 956–961.

14. Chan J. M., Jou R. M., Caroll P. R., "The relative impact and future burden of prostate cancer in the United States," *J. Urol.*, 2004, 172, pp. S13–S16; discussion p. S17.

15. Swagerty D. L. Jr., et al., "Lactose intolerance."

16. Ahn J., Albanes D., Peters U., Schatzkin A., Lim U., Freedman M., Chatterjee N., Andriole G. L., Leitzmann M. F., Hayes R. B., "Dairy products, calcium intake, and risk of prostate cancer in the Prostate, Lung, Colorectal, and Ovarian Cancer Screening Trial," *Cancer Epidemiol. Biomarkers Prev.*, 2007, 16 (12), pp. 2623–2630.

17. Harvard University Health Services, "Calcium content of common foods in common portions," available at huhs.harvard.edu/assets/File/ourservices/service_Nutrition_Calciumcontentofcommonfoods.pdf (accessed July 28, 2014).

18. Kesse E., Boutron-Ruault M. C., Norat T., Riboli E., Clavel-Chapelon F.,

"Dietary calcium, phosphorus, vitamin D, dairy products and the risk of colorectal adenoma and cancer among French women of the E3N-EPIC prospective study," *Int. J. Cancer*, 2005, 117 (1), pp. 137–144.

19. Huncharek M., Muscat J., Kupelnick B., "Colorectal cancer risk and dietary intake of calcium, vitamin D, and dairy products: A meta-analysis of 26,335 cases from 60 observational studies," *Nutr. Cancer*, 2009, 61 (1), pp. 47–69.

20. Szilagyi A., Nathwani U., Vinokuroff C., Correa J. A., Shrier I., "Evaluation of relationships among national colorectal cancer mortality rates, genetic lactase non-persistence status, and per capita yearly milk and milk product consumption," *Nutr. Cancer*, 2006, 55 (2), pp. 151–156.

21. Wollowski I., et al. "Protective role of probiotics and prebiotics in colon cancer."

22 World Cancer Research Fund, *Food, Nutrition, Physical Activity, and the Prevention of Cancer: A Global Perspective* (Washington, D.C., American Institute for Cancer Research, 2007).

Chapter 6: Fruits and Vegetables

1. U.S. Department of Agriculture, *ChooseMyPlate.gov*, www.choosemyplate.gov.

2. World Cancer Research Fund, *Food, Nutrition, Physical Activity, and the Prevention of Cancer: A Global Perspective,* (Washington, D.C., American Institute for Cancer Research, 2007).

3. Leverve X., *Stress oxidant et antioxidants* [Oxidative stress and antioxidants], 49ᵉ JAND, 2009, available at http://www.jand.fr./opencms/export/sites/jand/data /documents/Xavier_LEVERVE.pdf (accessed March 23, 2010).

4. Fernandez-Panchon M. S., Villano D., Troncoso A. M., Garcia-Parrilla M. C., "Antioxidant activity of phenolic compounds: From *in vitro* results to *in vivo* evidence," *Crit. Rev. Food Sci. Nutr.*, 2008, 48 (7), pp. 649–671.

5. Roussel A. M., *Qui manque d'antioxydants et comment le savoir?* [Who is deficient in antioxidants and how to know it?], 49ᵉ JAND, 2009, available at http://www.institute-benjamin-delessert.net/export/sites/default/.content /media/documents/JABD/resumes-2009/ROUSSEL.pdf (accessed July 27, 2014).

6. EUFIC [European Food Information Council], *La Couleur des fruits et légumes et la santé* [Colors of fruits and vegetables and health], available at http://www

.eufic.org/article/fr/rid/la-coleur-des-fruits-legumes-et-sante (accessed March 20, 2010).

7. Ibid.

8. World Cancer Research Fund, *Food, Nutrition, Physical Activity, and the Prevention of Cancer.*

9. EUFIC, *La Couleur des fruits et légumes et la santé.*

10. Ibid.

11. Aprifel, *Les fiches nutritionnelles par produits-chou vert* [Green cabbage information sheet], available at http://www.aprifel.com/fiche-nutri-produit-chou-vert,59.html (accessed December 11, 2014).

12. Larsson S. C., Håkansson N., Näslund I., Bergkvist L., Wolk., A., "Fruit and vegetable consumption in relation to pancreatic cancer risk: A prospective study," *Cancer Epidemiol. Biomarkers Prev.*, 2006, 15 (2), pp. 301–305.

13. EUFIC, *La Couleur des fruits et légumes et la santé.*

14. Oaks B. M., Dodd K. W., Meinhold C. L., Jiao L., Church T. R., Stolzenberg-Solomon R. Z., "Folate intake, post-folic acid grain fortification, and pancreatic cancer risk in the Prostate, Lung, Colorectal, and Ovarian Cancer Screening Trial," *Am. J. Clin. Nutr.*, 2010, 91 (2), pp. 449–455.

15. Balder H. F., Vogel J., Jansen M. C., Weijenberg M. P., Van den Brandt P. A., Westenbrink S., Van der Meer R., Goldbohm R. A., "Heme and chlorophyll intake and risk of colorectal cancer in the Netherlands Cohort Study," *Cancer Epidemiol Biomarkers Prev.*, 2006, 15 (4), pp. 717–725.

16. Vogel J. de, Jonker-Termont D. S., Van Lieshout E. M., Katan M. B., Van der Meer R., "Green vegetables, red meat and colon cancer: Chlorophyll prevents the cytotoxic and hyperproliferative effects of haem in rat colon," *Carcinogenesis*, 2005, 26 (2), pp. 387–393.

17. Daswood R. H., "Chlorophylls as anticarcinogens," *Int. J. Oncol.*, 1997, 10 (4), pp. 721–727.

18. EUFIC, *La Couleur des fruits et légumes et la santé.*

19. Ibid.

20. World Cancer Research Fund, *Food, Nutrition, Physical Activity, and the Prevention of Cancer.*

21. Ibid.

22. Abu J., Batuwangala M., Herbert K., Symonds P., "Retinoic acid and retinoid receptors: Potential chemopreventive and therapeutic role in cervical cancer," *Lancet Oncol.*, 2005, 6 (9), pp. 712–720.

23. EUFIC, *La Couleur des fruits et légumes et la santé.*

24. Ibid.

25. World Cancer Research Fund, *Food, Nutrition, Physical Activity, and the Prevention of Cancer.*

26. EUFIC, *La Couleur des fruits et légumes et la santé.*

27. World Cancer Research Fund, *Food, Nutrition, Physical Activity, and the Prevention of Cancer.*

28. Ibid.

29. Ibid.

30. EUFIC, *La Couleur des fruits et légumes et la santé.*

31. Seeram N. P., Adams L. S., Zhang Y., Lee R., Sand D., Scheuller H. S., Heber D., "Blackberry, black raspberry, blueberry, cranberry, red raspberry, and strawberry extracts inhibit growth and stimulate apoptosis of human cancer cells *in vitro*," *J. Agric. Food Chem.*, 2006, 54 (25), pp. 9329–9339.

32. Mittal A., Elmets C. A., Katiyar S. K., "Dietary feeding of proanthocyanidins from grape seeds prevents photocarcinogenesis in SKH-1 hairless mice: Relationship to decreased fat and lipid peroxidation," *Carcinogenesis*, 2003, 24 (8), pp. 1379–1388.

33. Yi W., Fischer J., Krewer G., Akoh C. C., "Phenolic compounds from blueberries can inhibit colon cancer cell proliferation and induce apoptosis," *J. Agric. Food Chem.*, 2005, 53 (18), pp. 7320–7329.

34. EUFIC, *La Couleur des fruits et légumes et la santé.*

35. Yun J. M., Afaq F., Khan N., Mukhtar H., "Delphinidin, an anthocyanidin in pigmented fruits and vegetables, induces apoptosis and cell cycle arrest in human colon cancer HCT116 cells," *Mol. Carcinog.*, 2009, 48 (3), pp. 260–270.

36. Afaq F., Zaman N., Khan N., Syed D. N., Sarfaraz S., Zaid M. A., Mukhtar H., "Inhibition of epidermal growth factor receptor signaling pathway by delphinidin, an anthocyanidin in pigmented fruits and vegetables," *Int. J. Cancer*, 2008, 123 (7), pp. 1508–1515.

37. EUFIC, *La Couleur des fruits et légumes et la santé.*

38. Lin Y., Shi R., Wang X., Shen H. M., "Luteolin, a flavonoid with potential for cancer prevention and therapy," *Curr. Cancer Drug Targets*, 2008, 8 (7), pp. 634–646.

39. EUFIC, *La Couleur des fruits et légumes et la santé.*

40. Lin Y., et al., "Luteolin, a flavonoid with potential for cancer prevention and therapy."

41. Zhou Q., Yan B., Hu X., Li X. B., Zhang J., Fang J., "Luteolin inhibits invasion of prostate cancer PC3 cells through E-cadherin," *Mol. Cancer Ther.*, 2009, 8 (6), pp. 1684–1691.

42. Butler L. M., Wu A. H., Wang R., Koh W. P., Yuan J. M., Yu M. C., "A vegetable-fruit-soy dietary pattern protects against breast cancer among post-menopausal Singapore Chinese women," *Am. J. Clin. Nutr.*, 2010, 91 (4), pp. 1013–1019.

43. Armstrong B., Doll R., "Environmental factors and cancer incidence and mortality in different countries, with special reference to dietary practices," *Int. J. Cancer*, 1975, 15, pp. 617–631.

44. Food and Agriculture Organization of the United Nations (FAO), *INPhO: Compendium Chapter19 Soybeans 1.6 Consumer Preferences*, 2007, available at http://www.fao.org/inpho/content/compend/text/Ch19sec1_6.htm (accessed March 24, 2010).

45. Yan L., Spitznagel E. L., Bosland M. C., "Soy consumption and colorectal cancer risk in humans: A meta-analysis," *Cancer Epidemiol. Biomarkers Prev.*, 2010, 19 (1), pp. 148–158.

46. Nagata C., Takatsuka N., Kawakami N., Shimizu H., "A prospective cohort study of soy product intake and stomach cancer death," *Br. J. Cancer*, 2002, 87 (1), pp. 31–36.

47. Jacobsen B. K., Knutsen S. F., Fraser G. E., "Does high soy milk intake reduce prostate cancer incidence? The Adventist Health Study (United States)," *Cancer Causes Control*, 1998, 9 (6), pp. 553–557.

48. Kim H. Y., Yu R., Kim J. S., Kim Y. K., Sung M. K., "Antiproliferative crude soy saponin extract modulates the expression of IkappaBalpha, protein kinase C, and cyclooxygenase-2 in human colon cancer cells," *Cancer Lett.*, 2004, 210 (1), pp. 1–6.

49. Buteau-Lozano H., Velasco G., Cristofari M., Balaguer P., Perrot-Applanat M., "Xenoestrogens modulate vascular endothelial growth factor secretion in breast cancer cells through an estrogen receptor–dependent mechanism," *J. Endocrinol.*, 2008, 196 (2), pp. 399–412.

50. World Cancer Research Fund, *Food, Nutrition, Physical Activity, and the Prevention of Cancer.*

51. Aviello G., Abenavoli L., Borrelli F., Capasso R., Izzo A. A., Lembo F., Romano B., Capasso F., "Garlic: Empiricism or science?" *Nat. Prod. Commun.*, 2009, 4 (12), pp. 1785–1796.

52. World Cancer Research Fund, *Food, Nutrition, Physical Activity, and the Prevention of Cancer.*

53. Ibid.

54. Ibid.

55. Health Canada, *Nitrate/Nitrate*, June 1987, available at http://www.hc-sc .gc.ca./ewh-semt/pubs/water-eau/nitrate_nitrite/index-eng.php (accessed March 25, 2010).

56. Société canadienne du cancer, *Concentrations de résidus de pesticides dans les aliments* [Concentrations of pesticide residue in foods], 2007–2011, available at http://www.mapaq.gouv.qc.ca/SiteCollectionDocuments/Publications/Resi dus_pesticides_fruits_legumesWEB.pdf (accessed April 16, 2014).

57. EWG, *Shopper's Guide to Pesticides in Produce*, 2014, from www.ewg.org (accessed March 3, 2014).

58. Environmental Working Group, (EWG), *People Can Reduce Pesticide Exposure by 80 Percent through Smart Shopping and Using the Guide*, 2009, available at: http://www.ewg.org/news-releases/2009/03/10/EWG-updates-Pesticide-Shoppers-Guide (accessed March 25, 2010).

59. EWG, *Shopper's Guide to Pesticides in Produce*, 2013, from www.ewg.org.

60. U.S. Department of Agriculture, *Pesticide Data Program: Annual Summary, Calendar Year 2007* (Washington, D.C., USDA, 2008), p. 22.

61. Société canadienne du cancer, *Concentrations de résidus de pesticides dans les aliments.*

Chapter 7: Fats and Cooking Methods

1. Shields P. G., Xu G. X., Blot W. J., Fraumeni J. F. Jr., Trivers G. E., Pellizzari E. D., Qu Y. H., Gao Y. T., Harris C. C., "Mutagens from heated Chinese and US cooking oils," *J. Natl. Cancer Inst.*, 1995, 87 (11), pp. 836–841.

2. Yu I. T., Chiu Y. L., Au J. S., Wong T. W., Tang J. L., "Dose-response relationship between cooking fumes exposures and lung cancer among Chinese nonsmoking women," *Cancer Res.*, 2006, 66 (9), pp. 4961–4967.

3. PNNS [French Nutrition and Health Program], *Matières grasses: à limiter. Bien les choisir pour vraiment en profiter* [Fat: reduce. Make good choices to truly do well], available at http://www.mangerbouger.fr/bien-manger/que-veut-dire -bien-manger-127/les-9-reperes/matieres-grasses-a-limiter.html (accessed April 16, 2014).

4. ANSES, *Les apports nutritionnels conseillés* [Nutritional intake advice]. January 30, 2014, available at https://www.anses.fr/fr/content/les-apports-nutritionnels -conseill%C3%A9s (accessed April 16, 2014).

5. AFSSA [French Food Safety Agency], *French Food Composition Table: Table CIQUAL 2012*, available at http://pro.anses.fr/TableCIQUAL/ (accessed February 20, 2014).

6. U.S. Department of Agriculture, (USDA), National Nutrient Database for Standard Reference, Release 25. References used: Butter, without salt (01145), Goose fat (04576), Margarine, regular, 80% fat, composite, tub, without salt (04618), Lard (04002), Peanut Oil (04042).

7. USDA, National Nutrient Database for Standard Reference, Release 25. References used: Peanut Oil, salad or cooking (04042), Olive Oil, salad or cooking (04053), Canola Oil, (04582), Walnut, Oil (04428), Grapeseed Oil (04517), Soybean oil, salad or cooking (04044), Sunflower oil, linoleic (approx. 65%) (04506), Oil, corn, peanut, and olive (44005).

8. World Cancer Research Fund, *Food, Nutrition, Physical Activity, and the Prevention of Cancer: A Global Perspective* (Washington, D.C., American Institute for Cancer Research, 2007).

9. Ibid.

10. Ibid.

11. Pouyat-Leclère J., Birlouez I., *Cuisson et Santé. Guide des bonnes pratiques de cuisson pour une alimentation plus saine* [Cooking and health. A guide to cooking good practice for healthier eating] (Monaco, Calif. Alpen, 2005).

12. MacLean C. H., Newberry S. J., Mojica W. A., Khanna P., Issa A. M., Suttorp M. J., Lim Y. W., Traina S. B., Hilton L., Garland R., Morton S. C., "Effects of omega-3 fatty acids on cancer risk: A systematic review," *JAMA*, 2006, 295 (4), pp. 403–415.

13. Sanchez-Muniz F. J., "Oils and fats: Changes due to culinary and industrial processes," *Int. J. Vitam. Nutr. Res.*, 2006, 76 (4), pp. 230–237.

14. Warner K., "Impact of high-temperature food processing on fats and oils," *Adv. Exp. Med. Biol.*, 1999, 459, pp. 67–77.

15. Culinary Institute of America, *The New Professional Chef* (New York, John Wiley & Sons, 1996).

16. International Agency for Research on Cancer, (IARC), *Monographs on the Evaluation of Carcinogenic Risks to Humans*, available at http://monographs.iarc .fr/CENG/Classicication/index.php (accessed April 16, 2014).

17. DGCCRF [French Directorate General for Competition, Consumer Affairs and Repression of Fraud], *Qualite des huiles de friture* [Quality of cooking oils], 2001, available at http://www.dgccrf.bercy.gouv.fr/fonds_documentaire /dgccrf/04_dossiers/consommation/controles_alimentaires/actions/friture 0902.htm (accessed March 19, 2010).

18. Shields P. G., Xu G. X., Blot W. J., Fraumeni J. F. Jr., Trivers G. E., Pellizzari E. D., Qu Y. H., Gao Y. T., Harris C. C., "Mutagens from heated Chinese and US cooking oils," *J. Natl. Cancer Inst.*, 1995, 87 (11), pp. 836–841.

19. Lee C. H., Yang S. F., Peng C. Y., Li R. N., Chen Y. C., Chan T. F., Tsai E. M., Kuo F. C., Huang J. J., Tsai H. T., Hung Y. H., Huang H. L., Tsai S., Wu M. T., "The precancerous effect of emitted cooking oil fumes on precursor lesions of cervical cancer," *Int. J. Cancer*, December 9, 2009, epub.

20. Metayer C., Wang Z., Kleinerman R. A., Wang L., Brenner A. V., Cui H., Cao J., Lubin J. H., "Cooking oil fumes and risk of lung cancer in women in rural Gansu, China," *Lung Cancer*, 2002, 35 (2), pp. 111–117.

21. Ibid.

22. Lin S. Y., Tsai S. J., Wang L. H., Wu M. F., Lee H., "Protection by quercetin against cooking oil fumes–induced DNA damage in human lung adenocarcinoma CL-3 cells: Role of COX-2," *Nutr. Cancer*, 2002, 44 (1), pp. 95–101.

23. IARC, *Monographs on the Evaluations of Carcinogenic Risks to Humans*.

24. AFSSA, *Acrylamide: point d'information n°2*, 2003 [Acrylamide: point of information no. 2], available at: http://www.afssa.fr/Documents/RCCP2002sa0300. pdf (accessed March 19, 2010).

25. Health Canada, *Acrylamide levels in selected Canadian foods*, 2009, available

at http://www.hc-sc.gc.ca/fn-an/security/chem.-chim/food-aliment/acrylamide /acrylamide_level-acrylamide_niveau-eng.php (accessed March 19, 2010).

26. European Food Safety Authority (EFSA), *Acrylamide*, 2010, available at http:// www.efsa.europa.eu/fr/contamtopics/topic/acrylamide.htm (accessed March 19, 2010).

27. Mottram D. S., Wedzicha B. L., Dodson A. T., "Acrylamide is formed in the Maillard reaction," *Nature*, 2002, 419 (6906), pp. 448–449.

28. AFSSA, *Acrylamide*.

29. Food and Drug Administrations, *Survey Data on Acrylamide in Food: Total Diet Study Results*, "Table 4: Acrylamide Levels in Food Sampled for the 2006 Total Diet Study." October 2006, available at http://www.fda.gov/Food/Food borneillnessContaminants/ChemicalContaminants/ucm053566.htm #table 4 (accessed January 16, 2013).

30. Ibid.

31. Ibid.

32. Ibid.

33. American Cancer Society, *A Backyard Chief's Guide to Healthier Grilling*, July 10, 2010, available at http://www.cancer.org/cancer/news/features/a-backyard -chefs-guide-to-healthy-grilling (accessed January 21, 2012).

34. AFFSA, *Étude individuelle nationale des consommations alimentaires 2* [National Individual Study of Food Consumption 2] *(INCA 2) 2006–2007*, 2009 available at www.anses.fr/Documents/PASER-Ra-INCA2.pdf (accessed December 11, 2014).

Chapter 8: Sugars and Sugar Products

1. N'Diaye C. (sld.), *La gourmandise. Délices d'un péché* [Being fond of food. The delights of a sin] (Paris, Editions Autrement, Série Mutations/mangeurs, no. 140, 1993).

2. Guy-Grand B., "Les sucres dans l'alimentation: de quoi parle-t-on ?" [Sugars in diet: What are we talking about?], *Cah Nutr. Diét.*, 2008, hors-série 2.

3. World Cancer Research Fund, *Food, Nutrition, Physical Activity, and the Pre-*

vention of Cancer: A Global Perspective (Washington, D.C., American Institute for Cancer Research, 2007).

4. USDA, National Nutrient Database for Standard Reference, Release 25.

5. AFSSA [French Food Safety Agency], *French Food Composition Table: Table CIQUAL 2012*, available at http://pro.anses.fr/TableCIQUAL/ (accessed February 20 2014).

6. Cezard J. P., Forgue-Lafitte M. E., Chamblier M. C., Rosselin G. E., "Growth promoting effect, biological activity, and binding of insulin in human intestinal cancer cells in culture," *Cancer Res.*, 1981, 41 (3), pp. 1148–1153.

7. Mauro L. M., Morelli C., Boterberg T., Bracke M. E., Surmacz E., "Role of the IGF1 receptor in the regulation of cell-cell adhesion: Implications in cancer development and progression," *J. Cell. Physiol.*, 2003, 194 (2), pp. 108–116.

8. Plymate S. R., Jones R. E., Matej L. A., Friedl K. E., "Regulation of sex hormone binding globulin (SHBG) production in Hep G2 cells by insulin," *Steroids*, 1988, 52 (4), pp. 339–340.

9. Silvera S. A. N., Rohan T. E., Jain M., Terry P. D., Howe G., Miller A., "Glycemic index, glycemic load, and pancreatic cancer risk (Canada)," *Cancer Causes Control*, 2005, 16 (4), pp. 431–436.

10. Augustin L. S., Franceschi S., Jenkins D., Kendall C., La Vecchia C., "Glycemic index in chronic disease: A review," *Eur. J. Clin. Nutr.*, 2002, 56 (11), pp. 1049–1071.

11. Cust A. E., Slimani N., Kaaks R., van Bakel M., Biessy C., Ferrari P., Laville M., Tjønneland A., Olsen A., Overvad K., Lajous M., Clavel-Chapelon F., Boutron-Ruault M.-C., Linseisen J., Rohrmann S., Nöthlings U., Boeing H., Pallli D., Sieri S., Panico S., Tumino R., Sacerdote C., Skeie G., Engeset D., Gram I. T., Quirós J. R., Jakszyn P., Sánchez M. J., Larrañaga N., Navarro C., Ardanaz E., Wirfält E., Berglund G., Lundin E., Hallmans G., Bueno-de-Mesquita H. B., Du H., Peeters P. H. M., Bingham S., Khaw K.-T., Allen N. E., Key T. J., Jenab M., Riboli E., "Dietary carbohydrates, glycemic index, glycemic load, and endometrial cancer risk within the European Prospective Investigation into Cancer and Nutrition cohort," *Am. J. Epidemiol.*, 2007, 166 (8), pp. 912–923.

12. Larsson S., Bergkvist L., Wolk A., "Glycemic load, glycemic index and breast cancer risk in a prospective cohort of Swedish women," *Int. J. Cancer*, 2009, 125, pp. 153–157.

13. Lajous M., Boutron-Ruault M. C., Fabre A., Clavel-Chapelon F., Romieu Y., "Carbohydrate intake, glycemic index, glycemic load, and risk of postmenopausal breast cancer in a prospective study of French women," *Am. J. Clin. Nutr.*, 2008, 87 (5), pp. 1384–1391.

14. Mulholland H. G., Murray L. J., Cardwell C. R., Cantwell M. M., "Glycemic index, glycemic load, and risk of digestive tract neoplasms: A systematic review and meta-analysis," *Am. J. Clin. Nutr.*, 2009, 89 (2), pp. 568–576.

15. Michaud D. S., Fuchs C. S., Liu S., Willett W. C., Colditz G. A., Giovannucci E., "Dietary glycemic load, carbohydrate, sugar, and colorectal cancer risk in men and women," *Cancer Epidemiol. Biomarkers Prev.* 2005, 14 (1), pp. 138–147.

16. Mulholland H. G., et al. "Glycemic index, glycemic load, and risk of digestive tract neoplasms."

17. Howarth N. C., Murphy S. P., Wilkens L. R., Henderson B. E., Kolonel L. N., "The association of glycemic load and carbohydrate intake with colorectal cancer risk in the Multiethnic Cohort Study," *Am. J. Clin. Nutr.*, 2008, 88 (4), pp. 1074–1082.

18. American Cancer Society, *Prevention and Early Detection: Aspartame*, 2007, available at http://www.cancer.org/docroot/PED/content/PED_1_3X_Aspartame.asp (accessed March 17, 2010).

19. American Cancer Society, *Guidelines on Nutrition and Physical Activity for Cancer Prevention*, available at www.cancer.org/acs/groups/cid/documents/webcontent-002577-pdf.pdf (accessed March 17, 2010).

20. American Cancer Society, *Prevention and Early Detection*.

21. Phillips K. M., Carlsen M. H., Blomhoff R., "Total antioxidant content of alternatives to refined sugar," *J. Am. Diet. Assoc.*, 2009, 109 (1), pp. 64–71.

Chapter 9: What Should We Drink?

1. CNRS [French National Center for Scientific Research], *Découvrir l'eau. L'eau dans l'organisme* [Discovering water. Water in the body], available at: http://www.cnrs.fr/cw/dossiers/doseau/decouv/usages/eauOrga.html (accessed March 17, 2010).

2. World Health Organization (WHO), *Selon un nouveau rapport, la réalisation des cibles en matière d'assainissement et d'eau potable serait compromise* [According to

a recent report, achieving safe water and drinking water goals will be compromised], press release, 2006, available at http://www.who.int/mediacentre/news/releases/2006/pr47/fr/index.html (accessed March 17, 2010).

3. WHO, *Water Sanitation and Health: Health through Safe Drinking Water and Basic Sanitation*, available at http://www.who.int/water_sanitation_health/mdg1/en/index.html (accessed March 17, 2010).

4. U.S. Environmental Protection Agency (EPA), *Fiscal Year 2010 Drinking Water and Ground Water Statistics*, June 2011, available at water.epa.gov/scitech/datait/databases/drink/sdwisfed/upload/new_fiscal-year-2010-drinking-water-and-ground-water-statistics.pdf (accessed May 12, 2014).

5. Ibid.

6. Ibid.

7. EPA, *How to Access Local Drinking Water Information*, available at http://www.epa.gov/drink/local (accessed July 27, 2014).

8. Ibid.

9. World Cancer Research Fund, *Food, Nutrition, Physical Activity, and the Prevention of Cancer: A Global Perspective* (Washington, D.C., American Institute for Cancer Research, 2007).

10. Olson E. D., "Bottled water contamination: An overview of NRDC's and others' surveys," in *Bottled Water: Pure Drink or Pure Hype?*, April 1999, available at http://www.nrdc.org/water/drinking/bw/chap3.asp (accessed March 17, 2010).

11. DU Nutrition, Université de Paris Descartes.

12. Environmental Working Group (EWG), "Big City Water Ratings," 2009, available at www.ewg.org/tap-water/rating-big-city-water.php (accessed July 28, 2014).

13. Ibid.

14. Environmental Working Group (EWG), "EWG's Top-Rated and Lowest-Rated Water Utilities—2009," available at www.ewg.org/tap-water (accessed July 28, 2014).

15. World Cancer Research Fund, *Food, Nutrition, Physical Activity, and the Prevention of Cancer*.

16. Ibid.

17. Fakhry C., Gillison M. L., "Clinical implications of human papillomavirus in head and neck cancers," *J. Clin. Oncol.*, 2006, 24 (17), pp. 2606–2611.

18. World Cancer Research Fund, *Food, Nutrition, Physical Activity, and the Prevention of Cancer.*

19. Ibid.

20. Adrian M., Jeandet P., Brevil A. C., Levite D., Debord S., Bessis R., "Assay of resveratrol and derivative stillbenes in wines by direct inspection high performance liquid chromatography," *Am. J. Enol. Vitic.*, 2000, 51, pp. 37–41.

21. Sun W., Wang W., Kim J., Keng P., Yang S., Zhang H., Liu C., Okunieff P., Zhang L., "Anticancer effect of resveratrol is associated with induction of apoptosis via a mitochondrial pathway alignment," *Adv. Exp. Med. Biol.*, 2008, 614, pp. 179–186.

22. Aprifel, *Rôle bénéfique des polyphénols et du resvératrol du vin* [The beneficial role of polyphenols and resveratrol in wine], 2001, available at http://www.caducee .net/dossierspecialises/nutrition/aprifel/polyphenols-resveratrol.asp (accessed March 17, 2010).

23. Renaud S., Lorgeril M. de, "Wine, alcohol, platelets, and the French paradox for coronary heart disease," *Lancet*, 1992, 339 (8808), pp. 1523–1526.

24. Brisdelli F., D'Andrea G., Bozzi A., "Resveratrol: A natural polyphenol with multiple chemopreventive properties," *Curr. Drug Metab.*, 2009, 10 (6), pp. 530–546.

25. Athar M., Back J. H., Kopelovich L., Bickers D. R., Kim A. L., "Multiple molecular targets of resveratrol: Anti-carcinogenic mechanisms," *Arch. Biochem. Biophys.*, 2009, 486 (2), pp. 95–102.

26. Yusuf N., Nasti T. H., Meleth S., Elmets C. A. "Resveratrol enhances cell-mediated immune response to DMBA through TLR4 and prevents DMBA-induced cutaneous carcinogenesis," *Mol. Carcinog.*, 2009, 48 (8), pp. 713–723.

27. Seeni A., Takahashi S., Takeshita K., Tang M., Sugiura S., Sato S. Y., Shirai T., "Suppression of prostate cancer growth by resveratrol in the transgenic rat for adenocarcinoma of prostate (TRAP) model," *Asian Pac. J. Cancer Prev.*, 2008, 9 (1), pp. 7–14.

28. Sengottuvelan M., Deeptha K., Nalini N., "Influence of dietary resveratrol on early and late molecular markers of 1,2-dimethylhydrazine-induced colon carcinogenesis," *Nutrition*, 2009, 25 (11–12), pp. 1169–1176.

29. Ding X. Z., Adrian T. E., "Resveratrol inhibits proliferation and induces apoptosis in human pancreatic cancer cells," *Pancreas*, 2002, 25 (4), pp. 71–76.

30. Woodall C. E., Li Y., Liu Q. H., Wo J., Martin R. C., "Chemoprevention of metaplasia initiation and carcinogenic progression to esophageal adenocarcinoma by resveratrol supplementation," *Anticancer Drugs*, 2009, 20 (6), pp. 437–443.

31. AFSSA [French Food Safety Agency], *French Food Composition Table: Table CIQUAL 2012*, available at http://www.afssa.fr/TableCIQUAL/ (accessed February 20, 2014).

32. Ibid.

33. French General Health Directorate, *Cancer de la peau. Mélanome* [Skin cancer. Melanoma], 2003, available at http://www.sante.gouv.fr/htm/dossiers/losp/34cancer_peau.pdf (accessed March 18, 2010).

34. AFSSET [French Agency for Health Security of the Environment and Work], *Rayonnement ultraviolet* [Ultraviolet radiation], available at http://www.anses.fr/fr/glossaires/656 accessed July 27, 2014).

35. Sayre R. M., Dowdy J. C., "The increase in melanoma: Are dietary furocoumarins responsible?" *Med. Hypotheses*, 2008, 70 (4), pp. 855–859.

36. Feskanich D., Willett W. C., Hunter D. J., Colditz G. A., "Dietary intakes of vitamins A, C, and E and risk of melanoma in two cohorts of women," *Br. J. Cancer*, 2003, 88 (9), pp. 1381–1387.

37. Malik A., Afaq F., Sarfaraz S., Adhami V. M., Syed D. N., Mukhtar H., "Pomegranate fruit juice for chemoprevention and chemotherapy of prostate cancer," *Proc. Natl. Acad. Sci. U. S. A.*, 2005, 102 (41), pp. 14813–14818.

38. Pantuck A. J., Leppert J. T., Zomorodian N., Aronson W., Hong J., Barnard R. J., Seeram N., Liker H., Wang H., Elashoff R., Heber D., Aviram M., Ignarro L., Belldegrun A., "Phase II study of pomegranate juice for men with rising prostate-specific antigen following surgery or radiation for prostate cancer," *Clin. Cancer Res.*, 2006, 12 (13), pp. 4018–4026.

39. Zhang Y., Seeram N. P., Heber D., Chen S., Adams L. S., "Pomegranate ellagitannin-derived compounds exhibit antiproliferative and antiaromatase activity in breast cancer cells *in vitro*," *Cancer Prev. Res.* (Philadelphia, Penn.), 2010, 3 (1), pp. 108–113.

40. Khan G. N., Gorin M. A., Rosenthal D., Pan Q., Bao L. W., Wu Z. F., Newman R. A., Pawlus A. D., Yang P., Lansky E. P., Merajver S. D., "Pomegranate

fruit extract impairs invasion and motility in human breast cancer," *Integr. Cancer Ther.*, 2009, 8 (3), pp. 242–253.

41. Seeram N. P., Adams L. S., Henning S. M., Niu Y., Zhang Y., Nair M. G., Heber D., "*In vitro* antiproliferative, apoptotic and antioxidant activities of punicalagin, ellagic acid and a total pomegranate tannin extract are enhanced in combination with other polyphenols as found in pomegranate juice," *J. Nutr. Biochem.*, 2005, 16 (6), pp. 360–367.

42. Gil M. I., Tomás-Barberán F. A., Hess-Pierce B., Holcroft D. M., Kader A. A., "Antioxidant activity of pomegranate juice and its relationship with phenolic composition and processing," *J. Agric. Food Chem.*, 2000, 48 (10), pp. 4581–4589.

43. Khan N., Afaq K., Kweon M. H., Kim K., Mukhtar H., "Oral consumption of pomegranate fruit extract inhibits growth and progression of primary lung tumors in mice," *Cancer Res.*, 2007, 67 (7), pp. 3475–3482.

44. Gil M. I., et al., "Antioxidant activity of pomegranate juice and its relationship with phenolic composition and processing."

45. Khan N., et al., "Oral consumption of pomegranate fruit extract inhibits growth and progression of primary lung tumors in mice."

46. Pantuck A. J., et al. "Phase II study of pomegranate juice for men with rising prostate-specific antigen following surgery or radiation for prostate cancer."

47. Gil M. I., et al. "Antioxidant activity of pomegranate juice and its relationship with phenolic composition and processing."

48. MacMahon B., Yen S., Trichopoulos D., Warren K., Nardi G., "Coffee and cancer of the pancreas," *N. Engl. J. Med.*, 1981, 304 (11), pp. 630–633.

49. Nkondjock A., "Coffee consumption and the risk of cancer: An overview," *Cancer Lett.*, 2008, 277 (2), pp. 121–125.

50. World Cancer Research Fund, *Food, Nutrition, Physical Activity, and the Prevention of Cancer.*

51. Pelucchi C., Tavani A., La Vecchia C., "Coffee and alcohol consumption and bladder cancer," *Scand. J. Urol. Nephrol.*, 2008, 218, suppl., pp. 37–44.

52. Baker J. A., Beehler G. P., Sawant A. C., Jayaprakash V., McCann S. E., Moysich K. B., "Consumption of coffee, but not black tea, is associated with decreased risk of premenopausal breast cancer," *J. Nutr.*, 2006, 136 (1), pp. 166–171.

53. Nkondjock A., Ghadirian P., Kotsopoulos J., Lubinski J., Lynch H., Kim-Sing C., Horsman D., Rosen B., Isaacs C., Weber B., Foulkes W., Ainsworth P., Tung N., Eisen A., Friedman E., Eng C., Sun P., Narod S. A., "Coffee consumption and breast cancer risk among BRCA1 and BRCA2 mutation carriers," *Int. J. Cancer*, 2006, 118 (1), pp. 103–107.

54. Shanafelt T. D., Lee Y. K., Call T. G., Nowakowski G. S., Dingli D., Zent C. S., Kay N. E., "Clinical effects of oral green tea extracts in four patients with low grade B-cell malignancies," *Leuk. Res.*, 2006, 30 (6), pp. 707–712.

55. Tsao A. S., Liu D., Martin J., Tang X. M., Lee J. J., El-Naggar A. K., Wistuba I., Culotta K. S., Mao L., Gillenwater A., Sagesaka Y. M., Hong W. K., Papadimitrakopoulou V., "Phase II randomized, placebo-controlled trial of green tea extract in patients with high-risk oral premalignant lesions," *Cancer Prev. Res.* (Philadelphia, Penn), 2009, 2 (11), pp. 931–941.

56. World Cancer Research Fund, *Food, Nutrition, Physical Activity, and the Prevention of Cancer*.

Chapter 10: Dietary Supplements and Nutrients

1. Food and Drug Administration, "Draft guidance for industry: Dietary supplements: New dietary ingredient notifications and related issues," 79 *Federal Register* 39111, July 5, 2011.

2. Gahche J., Bailey R., Burt V., Hughes J., Yetley E., Dwyer J., Picciano M. F., McDowell M., Sempos C., *Dietary Supplement Use among U.S. Adults Has Increased since NHANES III (1988–1994)* National Center for Health Statistics (NCHS) Data Brief, No. 61, April 2011, available at www.cdc.gov/nchs/data /databriefs/db61.pdf (accessed May 12, 2014).

3. Picciano M. F., Dwyer J. T., Radimer K. L., Wilson D. H., Fisher K. D., Thomas P. R., Yetley E. A., Moshfegh A. J., Levy P. S., Nielsen S. J., Marriott B. M., "Dietary supplement use among infants, children, and adolescents in the United States, 1999–2002," *Arch. Pediatr. Adolesc. Med.* 2007, 161 (10), pp. 978–985.

4. Ferrucci L. M., McCorkle R., Smith T., Stein K. D., Cartmel B., "Factors related to the use of dietary supplements by cancer survivors," *J. Altern. Complement. Med.*, 2009, 15 (6), pp. 637–680.

5. Cassileth B. R., Heitzer M., Wesa K., "The public health impact of herbs and nutritional supplements," *Pharm. Biol.*, 2009, 47 (8), pp. 761–767.

6. Kimura Y., Ito H., Ohnishi R., Hatano T., "Inhibitory effects of polyphenols on human cytochrome P450 3A4 and 2C9 activity," *Food Chem. Toxicol.*, 2009, 48 (1), pp. 429–435.

7. Goodman G. E., Thornquist M. D., Balmes J., Cullen M. R., Meyskens F. L. Jr., Omenn G. S., Valanis B., Williams J. H. Jr., "The Beta-Carotene and Retinol Efficacy Trial: Incidence of lung cancer and cardiovascular disease mortality during 6-year follow-up after stopping beta-carotene and retinol supplements," *J. Natl. Cancer Inst.*, 2004, 96 (23), pp. 1743–1750.

8. Virtamo J., Pietinen P., Huttunen J. K., Korhonen P., Malila N., Virtanen M. J., Albanes D., Taylor P. R., Albert P., ATBC Study Group, "Incidence of cancer and mortality following alpha-tocopherol and beta-carotene supplementation: A postintervention follow-up," *JAMA*, 2003, 290 (4), pp. 476–485.

9. Cook N. R., Le I. M., Manson J. E., Buring J. E., Hennekens C. H., "Effects of beta-carotene supplementation on cancer incidence by baseline characteristics in the Physicians' Health Study (United States)," *Cancer Causes Control*, 2000, 11 (7), pp. 617–626.

10. Lee I. M., Cook N. R., Manson J. E., Buring J. E., Hennekens C. H., "Betacarotene supplementation and incidence of cancer and cardiovascular disease: The Women's Health Study," *J. Natl. Cancer Inst.*, 1999, 91 (24), pp. 2102–2106.

11. De Klerk N. H., Musk A. W., Ambrosini G. L., Eccles J. L., Hansen J., Olsen N., Watts V. L., Lund H. G., Pang S. C., Beilby J., Hobbs M. S., "Western Perth asbestos workers, vitamin A and cancer prevention II: Comparison of the effects of retinol and beta-carotene," *Int. J. Cancer*, 1998, 75 (3), pp. 362–367.

12. Hercberg S., Kesse-Guyot E., Druesne-Pecollo N., Touvier M., Favier A., Latino-Martel P., Briançon S., Galan P., "Incidence of cancers, ischemic cardiovascular diseases and mortality during 5-year follow-up after stopping antioxidant vitamins and minerals supplements: A post-intervention follow-up in the SU.VI.MAX Study," *Int. J. Cancer*, 2010, epub.

13. Meyer F., Galan P., Douville P., Bairati I., Kegle P., Bertrais S., Estaquio C., Hercberg S., "Antioxidant vitamin and mineral supplementation and prostate cancer prevention in the SU.VI.MAX trial," *Int. J. Cancer*, 2005, 116 (2), pp. 182–186.

14. Hercberg S., Ezzedine K., Guinot C., Preziosi P., Galan P., Bertrais S., Estaquio C., Briançon S., Favie A., Latreille, J., Malvy, D., "Antioxidant supplementation increases the risk of skin cancers in women but not in men," *J. Nutr.*, 2007, 137, pp. 2098–2105.

15. Omenn G. S., Goodman G. E., Thornquist M. D., Balmes J., Cullen M. R.,

Glass A., Keogh J. P., Meyskens F. L. Jr., Valanis B., Williams J. H. Jr., Barnhart S., Cherniack M. G., Brodkin C. A., Hammar S., "Risk factors for lung cancer and for intervention effects in CARET, the Beta-Carotene and Retinol Efficacy Trial," *J. Natl. Cancer Inst.*, 1996, 88 (21), pp. 1550–1559.

16. National Cancer Institute, *Selenium and Vitamin E Cancer Prevention Trial (SELECT)*, 2008, available at http://www.cancer.gov/newscenter/qa/2008/selectqa accessed July 27, 2014.

17. National Cancer Institute, *Questions and Answers*.

18. Nelson R. L., "Iron and colorectal cancer risk, human studies," *Nutr. Rev.*, 2001, 59, pp. 140–148.

19. Duffield-Lillico A. J., Dalkin B. L., Reid M. E., Turnbull B. W., Slate E. H., Jacobs E. T., Marshall J. R., Clark L. C., "Nutritional Prevention of Cancer Study Group. Selenium supplementation, baseline plasma selenium status and incidence of prostate cancer: An analysis of the complete treatment period of the Nutritional Prevention of Cancer Trial," *BJU Int.*, 2003, 91 (7), pp. 6008–6012.

20. Clark L. C., Combs G. F. Jr., Turnbull B. W., Slate E. H., Chalker D. K., Chow J., Davis L. S., Glover R. A., Graham G. F., Gross E. G., Krongrad A., Lesher J. L. Jr., Park H. K., Sanders B. B. Jr., Smith C. L., Taylor J. R., "Effects of selenium supplementation for cancer prevention in patients with carcinoma of the skin. A randomized controlled trial," *JAMA*, 1996, 276 (24), pp. 1957–1963.

21. Ibid.

22. World Cancer Research Fund, *Food, Nutrition, Physical Activity and the Prevention of Cancer. A Global Perspective* (Washington, D.C., American Institute for Cancer Research, 2007).

23. Ibid.

24. Forrest K. Y., Stuhldreher W. L., "Prevalence and correlates of vitamin D deficiency in US adults," *Nutr. Res.* 2011, 31 (1), pp. (1) 48–54.

25. Jenab M., Bueno-de-Mesquita H. B., Ferrari P., Van Duijnhoven F. J., Norat T., Pischon T., Jansen E. H., Slimani N., Byrnes G., Rinaldi S., Tjønneland A., Olsen A., Overvad K., Boutron-Ruault M. C., Clavel-Chapelon F., Morois S., Kaaks R., Linseisen J., Boeing H., Bergmann M. M., Tichopoulou A., Misirli G., Trichopoulus D., Berrino F., Vineis P., Panico S., Palli D., Tumino R., Ros M. M., Van Gils C. H., Peeters P. H., Brustad M., Lund E., Tormo M. J., Ardanaz E., Rodriguez L., Sánchez M. J., Dorronsoro M., Gonzalez C. A., Hallmans G., Palmqvist R., Roddam A., Key T. J., Khaw K. T., Autier P.,

Hainaut P., Riboli E., "Association between pre-diagnostic circulating vitamin D concentration and risk of colorectal cancer in European populations: A nested case-control study," *BMJ*, 2010, 340, pp. b5500.

26. Ahn J., Albanes D., Peters U., Schatzkin A., Lim U., Freedman M., Chatterjee N., Andriole G. L., Leitzmann M. F., Hayes R. B., "Prostate, lung, colorectal, and ovarian trial project team. Dairy products, calcium intake, and risk of prostate cancer in the Prostate, Lung, Colorectal, and Ovarian Cancer Screening Trial", *Cancer Epidemiol. Biomarkers Prev.*, 2007, 16 (12), pp. 2623–2630.

27. Ruhul Amin A. R. M., Kucuk O., Khuri F. R., Shin D. M., "Perspectives for cancer prevention with natural compounds," *J. Clin. Oncol.*, 2009, 27 (18).

28. Ibid.

29. Hussain M., Banerjee M., Sarkar F. H., Djuric Z., Pollak M. N., Deorge D., Fontana J., Chinni S., Davis J., Forman J., Wood D. P., Kucuk O., "Soy isoflavones in the treatment of prostate cancer," *Nutr. Cancer*, 2006, 106, pp. 1260–1268.

30. Ibid.

31. Pendleton J. M., Tan W. W., Anai S., Chang M., Hou W., Shiverick K. T., Rosser C. J., "Phase II trial of isoflavone in prostate–specific antigen recurrent prostate cancer after previous local theraphy," *BMC Cancer*, 2008, 8 (132).

32. Chao J. C., Chiang S. W., Wang C. C., Tsai Y. H., Wu M. S., "Hot water–extracted *Lycium barbarum* and *Rehmannia glutinosa* inhibit proliferation and induce apoptosis of hepatocellular carcinoma cells," *World J. Gastroenterol.*, 2006, 12 (28), pp. 4478–4484.

33. Luo Q., Li Z., Yan J., Zhu F., Xu R. J., Cai Y. Z., "*Lycium barbarum* polysaccharides induce apoptosis in human prostate cancer cells and inhibits prostate cancer growth in a xenograft mouse model of human prostate cancer," *J. Med. Food*, 2009, 12 (4), pp. 695–703.

34. Mao F., Xiao B., Jiang Z., Zhao J., Huang X., Guo J., "Anticancer effect of *Lycium barbarum* polysaccharides on colon cancer cells involves G0/G1 phase arrest," *J. Med. Oncol.*, 2010, epub.

35. Miao Y., Xiao B., Jiang Z., Guo Y., Mao F., Zhao J., Huang X., Guo J., "Growth inhibition and cell-cycle arrest of human gastric cancer cells by *Lycium barbarum* polysaccharide," *J. Med. Oncol.*, 2009, epub.

36. Li G., Sepkovic D. W., Bradlow H. L., Telang N. T., Wong G. Y., "*Lycium barbarum* inhibits growth of estrogen receptor positive human breast cancer

cells by favorably altering estradiol metabolism," *Nutr. Cancer*, 2009, 61 (3), pp. 408–414.

37. Chao J. C., Chiang S. W., Wang C. C., Tsai Y. H., Wu M. S., "Hot water–extracted *Lycium barbarum* and *Rehmannia glutinosa* inhibit proliferation and induce apoptosis of hepatocellular carcinoma cells," *World J. Gastroenterol.*, 2002, 12 (28), pp. 4478–4484.

38. Ruhul Amin A. R. M., Kucuk O., Khuri F. R., et al., "Perspectives for cancer prevention with natural compounds."

Chapter 11: Keeping Physically Active Keeps Us Healthy

1. Reeves G. K., Pirie K., Beral V., Green J., Spencer E., Bull D., "Cancer incidence and mortality in relation to body mass index in the million women study: Cohort study," *BMJ*, 2007, 335 (7630), pp. 1134.

2. Renehan A. G., Soerjomataram I., Tyson M., Egger M., Zwahlen M., Coebergh J. W., Buchan I., "Incident cancer burden attributable to excess body mass index in 30 European countries," *Int. J. Cancer*, 2010, 126 (3), pp. 692–702.

3. World Health Organization (WHO), *Media Centre: Obesity and Overweight*, 2006, available at http://www.who.int/mediacentre/factsheets/fs311/en/ (accessed July 27, 2014).

4. Ogden C. L., Carroll M. D., Kit B. K., Flegal K. M., *Prevalence of Obesity in the United States, 2009–2010*. NCHS Data Brief, No. 82 (Hyattsville, Md., National Center for Health Statistics, 2012).

5. Ibid.

6. Ibid.

7. Stone R. J., *Atlas of Skeletal Muscles*, William C. Brown, 3rd ed. (Dubuque, Iowa, William C. Brown, 1999).

8. Ogden C. L. Lamb M. M., Carroll M. D., Flegal K. M., *Obesity and Socioeconomic Status in Children: United States, 1988–1994 and 2005–2008*. NCHS Data Brief No. 51 (Hyattsville, Md., National Center for Health Statistics, 2010).

9. Wu Y., "Overweight and obesity in China," *BMJ*, 2006, 333 (7564), pp. 362–363.

10. Bray G. A., "The epidemic of obesity and changes in food intake: The fluoride hypothesis," *Physiol Behav.*, 2004, 82 (1), pp. 115–121.

11. Burdette H. L., Whitaker R. C., "Neighborhood playgrounds, fast food restaurants, and crime: Relationships to overweight in low-income preschool children," *Prev. Med.*, 2004, 38, pp. 57–63.

12. U. S. Department of Agriculture, *Agriculture Fact Book 2001–2002* (Washington, D.C., U.S. Government Printing Office, March 2003), available at www.usda.gov/factbook/2002factbook.pdf (accessed May 12, 2014).

13. Nielsen S. J., Popkin B. M., "Changes in beverage intake between 1977 and 2001," *Am. J. Prev. Med.* 2004, 27, (3), pp. 205–210.

14. Burdette H. L., Whitaker R. C., "Neighborhood playgrounds, fast food restaurants, and crime."

15. Ibid.

16. Marchhall S. J., Biddle S. J., Gorely T., Cameron N., Murdey I., "Relationships between media use, body fatness and physical activity in children and youth: A meta-analyses," *Int. J. Obes. Relat. Metab. Disord.*, 2004, 28 (10), pp. 1238–1246.

17. Von Kries R., Toschke A. M., Wurmser H., Sauerwald T., Koletzko B., "Reduced risk for overweight and obesity in 5- and 6-y-old children by duration of sleep—a cross-sectional study," *Int. J. Obes. Relat. Metab. Disord.*, 2002, 26 (5), p. 710–716.

18. Miles L., "Physical activity and health," *Nutri. Bull.*, 2007, 32 (4), pp. 314–363.

19. Courneya K. S., Karvinen K. H., Campbell K. L., Pearcey R. G., Dundas G., Capstick V., Tonkin K. S., "Associations among exercise, body weight, and quality of life in a population-based sample of endometrial cancer survivors," *Gynecol. Oncol.*, 2005, 97 (2), pp. 422–430.

20. Holmes M. D., Chen W. Y., Feskanich D., Kroenke C. H., Colditz G. A., "Physical activity and survival after breast cancer diagnosis," *JAMA*, 2005, 293 (20), pp. 2479–2486.

21. Pierce J. P., Stefanick M. L., Flatt S. W., Natarajan L., Sternfeld B., Madlensky L., Al-Delaimy W. K., Thomson C. A., Kealey S., Hajek R., Parker B. A., Newman V. A., Caan B., Rock C. L., "Greater survival after breast cancer in physically active women with high vegetable-fruit intake regardless of obesity," *J. Clin. Oncol.*, 2007, 25 (17), pp. 2345–2351.

22. Knols R., Aaronson N. K., Uebelhart D., Fransen J., Aufdemkampe G., "Physical exercise in cancer patients during and after medical treatment: A systematic review of randomized and controlled clinical trials," *J. Clin. Oncol.*, 2005, 23 (16), pp. 3830–3842.

23. Irwin M. L., Smith A. W., McTiernan A., Ballard-Barbash R., Cronin K., Gilliland F. D., Baumgartner R. N., Baumgartner K. B., Bernstein L., "Influence of pre- and postdiagnosis physical activity on mortality in breast cancer survivors: The Health, Eating, Activity, and Lifestyle Study," *J. Clin. Oncol.*, 2008, 26 (24), pp. 3958–3964.

24. Cramp F., Daniel J., "Exercise for the management of cancer-related fatigue in adults," *J. Clin. Oncol.*, Cochrane Database, 2008, rev. 2012. epub: online library.wiley.com/doi/10.1002/14651858.D006145.pub3/abstract

25. Holick C. N., Newcomb P. A., Trentham-Dietz A., Titus-Ernstoff L., Bersch A. J., Stampfer M. J., Baron J. A., Egan K. M., Willett W. C., "Physical activity and survival after diagnosis of invasive breast cancer," *Cancer Epidemiol. Biomarkers Prev.*, 2008, 17 (2), pp. 379–386.

26. Pierce J. P., et al. "Greater survival after breast cancer in physically active women with high vegetable-fruit intake regardless of obesity."

27. Knols R., et al. "Physical exercise in cancer patients during and after medical treatment."

28. Rennie M. J., "Exercise- and nutrient-controlled mechanisms involved in maintenance of the musculoskeletal mass," *Biochem. Soc. Trans.*, 2007, 35 (pt. 5), pp. 1302–1305.

29. Holmes M. D., et al., "Physical activity and survival after breast cancer diagnosis."

30. Pierce J. P., et al., "Greater survival after breast cancer in physically active women with high vegetable-fruit intake regardless of obesity."

31. Harris C. D., Watson K. B., Carlson S. A., Fulton J. E., Dorn J. M., Elam-Evans, L., "Adult participation in aerobic and muscle-strengthening physical activities—United States, 2011, *MMWR Weekly*, May 3, 2013, 62 (17), pp. 326–330, available at http://www.cdc.gov/mmwr/preview/mmwrhtml/ mm6217a2.htm?s_cid=mm6217a2_e (accessed July 27, 2014)

32. Holmes M. D., Chen W. Y., Feskanich D., Kroenke C. H., Colditz G. A., "Physical activity and survival after breast cancer diagnosis," *JAMA*, 2005, 293 (20), pp. 2479–2486.

33. Pierce J. P., Stefanick M. L., Flatt S. W., Natarajan L., Sternfeld B., Madlen-

sky L., Al-Delaimy W. K., Thomson C. A., Kealey S., Hajek R., Parker B. A., Newman V. A., Caan B., Rock C. L., "Greater survival after breast cancer in physically active women with high vegetable-fruit intake regardless of obesity," *J. Clin. Oncol.*, 2007, 25 (17), pp. 2345–2351.

34. Holick C. N., Newcomb P. A., Trentham-Dietz A., Titus-Ernstoff L., Bersch A. J., Stampfer M. J., Baron J. A., Egan K. M., Willett W. C., "Physical activity and survival after diagnosis of invasive breast cancer," *Cancer Epidemiol. Biomarkers Prev.*, 2008, 17 (2), pp. 379–386.

35. Haskell B., *The Compendium of Physical Activities*, available at http://www .prevention.sph.sc.edu/tools/docs/documents_compendium.pdf (accessed March 29, 2010).

36. Jeon J., Sato K., Niedzwiecki D., Ye X., Saltz L. B., Mayer R. J., Mowat R. B., Whittom R., Hantel A., Benson A., Wigler D. S., Atienza D., Messino M., Kindler H., Venook A., Fuchs C. S., Meyerhardt J. A., "Impact of physical activity after cancer diagnosis on survival in patients with recurrent colon cancer: Findings from CALGB 89803 Alliance," *Clin. Colorectal Cancer*, 2013, 12 (4), pp. 233–238.

Chapter 12: Anticancer Advice

1. Carlsen M. H., Halvorsen B. L., Holte K., Bøhn S. K., Dragland S., Sampson L., Willey C., Senoo H., Umezono Y., Sanada C., Barikmo I., Berhe N., Willett W. C., Phillips K. M., Jacobs D. R. Jr., Blomhoff R., "The total antioxidant content of more than 3,100 foods, beverages, spices, herbs and supplements used worldwide," *Nutr. J.*, 2010, 9 (3).

Conclusion

1. American Cancer Society, *Cancer Facts and Figures 2014*, available at http://www.cancer.org/research/cancerfactsstatistics/cancerfactsfigures2014/index (accessed July 27, 2014).

Your Anticancer Checklist

1. Ruhul Amin A. R. M., Kucuk O., Khuri F. R., Shin D. M., "Perspectives for cancer prevention with natural compounds," *J. Clin. Oncol.*, 2009, 27 (18).

Index

Page numbers in *italics* refer to tables.

Your Anticancer Checklist

....

• 5 golden rules to lower your risk of getting cancer

1. **Don't smoke.** Remember that tobacco is carcinogenic from the first cigarette you smoke.

2. **Eat a varied diet.** You can eat small amounts of everything. Eating certain potentially carcinogenic products too much and too often can be dangerous.

3. **Try different ways of cooking your food.** Steaming and stewing are far healthier ways to cook.

4. **Try to eat local, seasonal, and sustainably grown products.** Always choose products with the lowest-possible pesticide residue.

5. **Rebalance your energy input and output.** Be more physically active and reduce your calorie intake. Don't snack between meals. Exercise regularly.

• Your top-ten foods and habits— invaluable for cancer prevention

1. **Pomegranate juice.** Drink store-bought juice.

2. **Turmeric.** Go ahead and use it whenever you can.

3. **Green tea.** All green teas are excellent.

4. **Wine.** It's full of resveratrol, but you should only drink small amounts.

5. **Selenium.** It has been proved to prevent cancer. Seek advice from your pharmacist or family doctor.

6. **Tomatoes.** They are rich in lycopene. Opt for cooked tomatoes or tomato sauce or tomato juice.

7. **Dietary fiber.** It is very important, as prebiotics and then to speed along your digestion.

8. **Garlic and onions.** These are remarkable anticancer agents. Add them to your food whenever possible.

9. **Quercetin.** It is found in capers, lovage, cocoa, and hot chili peppers. It is excellent if you smoke.

10. **Physical exercise.** Find a sport that suits you and do it regularly.

• Products and habits you should avoid

1. **Salmon, swordfish, red tuna, halibut.** Don't eat too much of them.

2. **Milk, cheese, and yogurt.** These are excellent for women and children. Men over fifty should cut their intake down.

3. **Beta-carotene.** If you smoke, and also if you're an ex-smoker, avoid beta-carotene as it's harmful to your health. Bear this in mind if you tend to eat lots of mangoes, carrots, apricots, squash, peaches, pumpkin, and sweet potatoes.

4. **Vitamin E.** Men should be very careful with vitamin E, which is found in many of the multivitamin products sold both in drugstores and on the Internet—always check carefully.

5. **Spirits.** Drinking hard liquor on a regular basis can increase the risk of certain cancers. Never drink more than an average of 30 g (1 oz.) of pure ethanol a day.

6. **Keep a careful eye on your weight.** Watch your waistline. You can't ignore it any longer—this applies to both you and your children.

7. **Arsenic in drinking water, nitrites, and nitrates in water and some deli meats.** You should systematically avoid them.

8. **Blood in meat.** Drain the blood from your meat before cooking it.

9. **Fats rich in polyunsaturated fatty acids.** Avoid these, especially rapeseed, perilla, and hemp seed oil, and especially when heated to a high temperature.

10. **Grilling and cooking with a wok.** Only very occasionally should you cook like this at a very high temperature.

• Foods and their anticancer benefits or risks

FISH AND CRUSTACEANS	HEALTHY OR HARMFUL	CANCER RANKING
Battered, breaded fish	**Check which fish is used (often lean) and how it's cooked; palm oil common**	**Not at all good**
Cod, fresh	A lean fish; less contaminated than oily fish	Good
Crab	Often contaminated with heavy metals and PCBs	Exercise caution
Halibut	Often contaminated with heavy metals and PCBs	Exercise caution
Oysters	Rich in selenium	Good
Pollock	A lean fish; less contaminated than oily fish	Good
Salmon	Often contaminated with heavy metals and PCBs	Exercise caution
Salmon taramasalata	A high-energy food; high in fat and a source of omega-3 (depending on which oil is used)	Average
Sardines in sunflower oil	Poor omega-3 and omega-6 balance	Good
Sea urchins	Rich in iodine	Very good

(Table continues)

FISH AND CRUSTACEANS	HEALTHY OR HARMFUL	CANCER RANKING
Shrimp	Low in fat and little contamination	Very good
Smoked fish	High in salt and polycyclic aromatic hydrocarbon content	Not good
Sushi	High in polyunsaturated fatty acids but also often contaminated	Exercise caution
Tuna	Often contaminated with heavy metals and PCBs	Exercise caution, especially with red tuna

MEAT AND DELI MEATS	HEALTHY OR HARMFUL	CANCER RANKING
Beef	Try and get rid of the blood	No problem here
Blood sausage	High in heme iron	Not good
Chicken	Low in fat	Very good
Deli meats	High nitrate content (if industrially manufactured)	Exercise caution
Foie gras	Rich in iron	Good
Game	Fairly low in saturated fatty acids	Very good
Grilled meats	High polycyclic hydrocarbon content	Not good
Knackwurst	High in saturated fat, nitrites, and polyphosphates	Not very good
Lardons	High in salt and saturated fatty acids	Average
Offal	Often high hemoglobin content	In moderation
Pork	Fat content varies according to which cut you use	Don't eat the fat
Pork spareribs	Fatty, 23.6% fat content; the way it's cooked is carcinogenic	Not at all good
Rabbit	Useful source of polyunsaturated fatty acids	Very good
Steak tartare	Raw meat; rich in heme iron	Good

EGGS, MILK, AND CHEESE	HEALTHY OR HARMFUL	CANCER RANKING
Buttermilk	Rich in probiotics	Good
Cheese	Rich in calcium and vitamin D	Very good for children; good for women (check the fat content); men over 50 should limit intake
Cheese spread	High in saturated fatty acids and sodium	Not good
Condensed evaporated milk	High in calcium but watch out for the sugar	Not good
Cream	High in saturated fats	Men over 50 should cut down
Eggs	Contain two carotenoids: lutein and zeaxanthin	Very good
Heavy cream	Contains lactobacillus; can be high in fat	Average
Ice cream	High in fat, particularly saturated fats; high sugar content	Not good
Milk	Contains lactose, calcium, and vitamin D	Very good for children; good for women; men over 50 should limit intake
Yogurt	Contains living bacteria: probiotics	Good

(Table continues)

VEGETABLES, PULSES, STARCHY FOODS, ARO- MATIC HERBS, ALGAE	HEALTHY OR HARMFUL	CANCER RANKING
Agar-agar (red algae)	A gelling agent that may aid digestion	Average
Algae	Contain fucoxanthins and fucoid- ans with antioxidant	Very good
Aromatic herbs	Rich in antioxidants	Good
Artichokes	Contain inulin, a prebiotic	Very good
Arugula	Contains flavonoids, quercetin in particular, and carotenoids with antioxidant properties	Very good; eat plenty
Avocadoes	Rich in polyunsaturated fatty acids and B-group vitamins	Very good
Basil	Contains aromatic polyphenols with antioxidant properties and anti-inflammatory ursolic acid	Very good
Beets	A source of anthocyanins	Very good
Black olives	Rich in monounsaturated fatty acids; contain phenolic compounds	Good
Broccoli	Contains lots of folates, gluco- raphanin, isothiocyanates, and sulforaphane	Excellent
Brussels sprouts	Contain lots of indole com- pounds and isothiocyanates	Very good
Canned vegetables	A source of vitamins and min- erals (depending on the veg- etable); check the salt content carefully	Very good, espe- cially if tomatoes
Capers	Rich in quercetin	Excellent
Carrots	Rich in beta-carotene	Not that good
Cauliflower	Has almost no carotenoids; con- tains indole compounds	Very good

Celeriac (celery root)	Contains polyacetylenes that inhibit the growth of cancerous cells	Look out for pesticide residues
Chicory	Rich in inulin, a prebiotic	Watch out for acrylamide
Chilis	A source of quercetin	Very good
Chinese cabbage	A source of indole compounds and isothiocyanates	Very good
Coriander	Detoxifies heavy metals; contains aromatic polyphenols	Very good
Dill	A digestive stimulant	Very good
Eggplant	Rich in insoluble fiber	Good
Fennel	A low-calorie source of fiber and vitamin B9	Very good
French fries	High in fats and toxic compounds produced from the heated oil	Eat in moderation; use a good-quality oil
Garden peas	A source of lutein	Good
Garlic	Contains sulfur compounds	Extraordinary
Glutamate	A flavor enhancer used in place of salt (3 times less sodium than standard table salt), but possibly side effects: numbness in the neck, heart palpitations, etc.	Average
Green olives	Less fat than black olives (12.5 g vs. 30 g) and rich in monounsaturated fatty acids	Very good
Guacamole	Due to avocado, high in polyunsaturated fatty acids and B-group vitamins; make your own, as shop-bought guacamole is often very high in fat	Not bad
Hummus	Rich in complex carbohydrates, but usually high in fat and calories too, so best to make your own	Not very good
Lentils	A good source of plant proteins	Very good

(Table continues)

VEGETABLES, PULSES, STARCHY FOODS, ARO-MATIC HERBS, ALGAE	HEALTHY OR HARMFUL	CANCER RANKING
Lettuce	A source of lutein	Good
Lovage	Rich in flavonoids, and quercetin in particular	Very good
Mint	A good source of antioxidants; a painkiller, antiseptic, and digestive stimulant	Very good
Mushrooms	A low-calorie food containing lots of useful vitamins	Very good
Parsley	High in vitamin C and calcium	Very good
Parsnips	Contain apigenin, an antioxidant	Good
Potatoes	Complex carbohydrates and vitamin C in the skin; antioxidant properties	Good
Pumpkins	Rich in carotenoids	Good
Radishes, black	Contain sulfur compounds	Very good
Red cabbage	Contains anthocyanins	Good
Red kidney beans	A source of anthocyanins	Good
Red onions	A source of anthocyanins	Excellent
Rutabaga	A source of indole compounds	Good
Soy	Contains phytoestrogens	Good
Spinach	Rich in carotenoid and calcium	Good
Sunchokes	Contain inulin, which has a prebiotic action	Good
Sweet peppers	Contain bioflavonoids	Very good
Sweet potatoes	Contain complex carbohydrates and anthocyanins with antioxidant properties	Good
Tapenade (garlic plus black olives)	High in monounsaturated fatty acids but often high in fat	Not very good
Tofu	Contains phytoestrogens	Very good

Tomatoes	A source of lycopene	Excellent, especially for men
Tomatoes, dried in oil	Contain very bioavailable lycopene	Very good
Turnips	Contain indole compounds and sulfur heterosides	Very good
Vegetable stock	A source of vitamins, minerals, and antioxidants	Very good
Watercress	A source of indole compounds	Very good
White onions	Contain selenium with antioxidant properties	Excellent
Zucchini	Contain carotenoids	Very good

FRUITS, DRIED FRUIT, BERRIES	HEALTHY OR HARMFUL	CANCER RANKING
Almonds	Rich in vitamins	Good
Apples	Contain quercetin; high in fiber	Watch out for pesticides
Apricots	Rich in beta-carotene	Watch out for pesticides
Bananas	Rich in prebiotic fiber	Very good
Black currants	Contain anthocyanins	Excellent
Blackberries	A good source of anthocyanins	Very good
Blueberries	Contain tocotrienols and polyphenols with antioxidant properties	Very good; eat plenty
Cherries	A source of antioxidant anthocyanins and folates	Good
Cranberries	A source of antioxidant anthocyanins	Very good
Dried fruit	High sugar content	Average
Goji berries	Contain *Lycium barbarum*, a polysaccharide with antioxidant properties	Good
Grapefruit	A source of lycopene	Very good

(Table continues)

FRUITS, DRIED FRUIT, BERRIES	HEALTHY OR HARMFUL	CANCER RANKING
Grapes	Contain numerous polyphenols, including resveratrol	Very good
Guava	A source of lycopene	Good
Kiwi	A source of lutein	Very good
Mangoes	Rich in beta-carotene	Good
Melons	A source of lutein	Good
Nectarines	Contain bioflavonoids	Very good
Oranges	Rich in vitamin C and calcium	Good
Peaches	Rich in beta-carotene	Watch out for pesticides
Pears	Contain bioflavonoids	Watch out for pesticides
Pineapples	Contain bioflavonoids	Good
Plums	A good source of polyphenols	Good
Pomegranates	Contain ellagitannins, powerful antioxidants	Very good
Raspberries	Rich in anthocyanins; high mineral density	Good
Strawberries	Contain calcium and iron, as well as anthocyanins	Good
Walnuts	Contain omega-3	Very good
Watermelons	A source of lycopene	Very good

OILS, FATS, SAUCES	HEALTHY OR HARMFUL	CANCER RANKING
Brown butter	Contains lots of lipid peroxides	Not good
Cod-liver oil	Rich in omega-3	Good
Goose fat	High in saturated fatty acids	Good
Ketchup	High in lycopene	Good
Mayonnaise	Very high in fat	Not good
Olive oil	Mainly made up of monounsaturated fatty acids	Very good
Peanut oil	Mainly made up of monounsaturated fatty acids	Good

| Rapeseed oil | Contains polyunsaturated fatty acids; unstable if exposed to light and heat | Average |
| Sunflower oil | Contains polyunsaturated fatty acids; unstable if exposed to light and heat | Good |

SUGAR, SWEET-ENERS, SUGARY FOODS	HEALTHY OR HARMFUL	CANCER RANKING
Agave syrup	Low antioxidant power, equivalent to sugar	Nothing to offer
Aspartame	Tastes of sugar; zero calories	No problem
Butter croissant	High in saturated fats	Average
Candies	High in carbohydrates with no nutritional value	Not good
Doughnuts	High-fat content with toxic compounds from the heated oil	Not good
Fruit jelly / paste	High in sugar	Not good
Gingerbread	High in sugar	Not very good
Honey	Rich in fructose	Very good
Industrial-made croissant	Likely to contain trans fatty acids	Really not good
Jams	High in simple sugars without the goodness of the fruit (vitamins, fiber, and minerals)	Watch out for the calories
Potato chips	High acrylamide content	Very bad
Saccharose	High in calories (400 kcal/100 g)	No problem
Savory snacks	High acrylamide content	Not good
Sorbet	Often high in simple sugars; best to make your own sorbets using high-antioxidant fruit	Average; don't overdo it
Spreads	High fat and sugar concentration	Not very good
Stevia	High sweetening power	Not yet known

CEREALS	HEALTHY OR HARMFUL	CANCER RANKING
Barley	Rich in prebiotics	Very good
Brewers' yeast flakes	Rich in B-group vitamins (optimizing immunity)	Very good
Cereals	A risk of aflatoxins, but high in fiber	Not bad
Corn	A source of anthocyanins	Average
French toast	High acrylamide content	Not good
Linseed	Rich in lignans (have to be crushed before they can be eaten)	Good
Muesli	High in fiber; however, do check carefully as some brands contain lots of sugar	Not bad
Popcorn	Lots of complex carbohydrates and lipids; check how much salt and/or sugar is added; risk of acrylamide	Not at all good
Quinoa, seeds	Very high in magnesium and non-heme iron; a source of plant proteins; high in fiber	Very good
Rice	Rich in complex carbohydrates	Very good
Semolina, couscous, durum wheat	A good source of proteins and complex carbohydrates; always try to eat whole wheat as the outer husk contains antioxidant compounds	Good
Sesame seeds	High in protein and fiber	Very good
Spelt, seeds	High in fiber, plant proteins, and magnesium	Very good
White bread	Contains little fiber	Good
Whole-wheat bread	High in fiber with lots of complex carbohydrates	Very good

DRINKS	HEALTHY OR HARMFUL	CANCER RANKING
Apple juice	High in antioxidant polyphenols and pectin	Good
Bottled water	No pesticides, but some waters contain pollutants such as arsenic	Check before drinking
Carrot juice	High in beta-carotene	Not good
Coconut milk	High in fat (21%) and in saturated fatty acids (18%)	Average
Coffee	Anticarcinogenic properties seem due to it containing caffeine and polyphenols	Quite good
Fruit juice	High in sugar	Not good
Grape juice	Rich in flavonoids	Good
Hard liquor	High concentration of ethanol; drink in moderation	Less than 30g a day on average of pure ethanol
Kefir	Lots of probiotics	Good
Orange juice	Contains fucoumarins, suspected of playing a role in the upsurge of malignant melanoma	If you spend time in the sun or are at risk of melanoma, exercise caution
Pineapple juice	Contains bromelain, an enzyme that speeds up the digestion of fish and meat	Rather good
Pomegranate juice	Extremely rich in antioxidants; more than in wine or green tea	The best! Drink as much as you want!
Smoothie	Rich in antioxidants but also in simple sugars	Average
Sodas	Lots of simple sugars	Not good
Tap water	Depending on your area, may contain nitrates, pesticides, and/or arsenic	Check before drinking

(Table continues)

DRINKS	HEALTHY OR HARMFUL	CANCER RANKING
Tea	Contains epigallocatechin-3-gallate	Very good
Verbena tea, herbal tea	Try and use different types of herbal teas; calms digestion	Very good
Wine	Contains resveratrol, a powerful antioxidant with known anticancer properties	Very good, but drink in moderation

SPICES AND CONDIMENTS	HEALTHY OR HARMFUL	CANCER RANKING
Cinnamon	Anti-infective	Good
Dark chocolate	Contains antioxidants	Very good
Ginger	When fresh, contains lots of vitamin C	Excellent
Licorice	A digestive stimulant and a diuretic; raises blood pressure	Exercise caution
Mustard	Acidic	Good
Nutmeg	A digestive stimulant	Very good
Pepper	Contains piperine, which makes turmeric more effective	Excellent
Salt	Incriminated in some stomach cancers	In moderation
Soy sauce	Lots of salt	Not very good
Star anise	A digestive stimulant with antiseptic action	Very good
Turmeric	A yellow pigment containing curcumin	Excellent
Vanilla, extract	Antioxidant	Good
Vinegar	A digestive stimulant	No problem

• Recommended fish

MY RECOMMENDATIONS FOR WHAT YOU SHOULD AVOID OR EAT

	YOU SHOULD AVOID	YOU CAN ENJOY
Fish	Swordfish Marlin Red tuna Eels Salmon	Mackerel Anchovies Sardines Sea bream Bass Sole
Crustaceans and seafood	Spider crabs	Shrimp Cockles

• Recommended fruits and vegetables

TOP FRUITS AND VEGETABLES WITH THE MOST ANTIOXIDANTS

FRUITS		VEGETABLES	
FOOD	ANTIOXI-DANT SCORE (ORAC/100 G)	FOOD	ANTIOXI-DANT SCORE (ORAC/100 G)
Strawberries	1,540	Broccoli	890
Blackberries	2,036	Alfalfa	930
Blueberries	2,400	Brussels sprouts	980
Cherries	670	Eggplant	390
Kiwi	602	Onions	450
Oranges	750	Red peppers	710
Pink grapefruit	483	Kale	710
Plums	949	Spinach	1,260
Prunes	5,770	Beets	840
Raisins	2,830	Corn	400
Raspberries	1,220		
Red grapes	739		

• Simple ways to prevent cancer

1. Choose local, if possible organic or sustainably grown food products.
2. Wash your fruits and vegetables thoroughly, even using a little soap, before rinsing and peeling them.
3. It's best to peel your fruits and vegetables; you must remove the outer leaves from cabbage and lettuce.
4. Before cooking your meat, drain off the blood. Even if this might seem a little odd, rinse it under some water before preparing it.

• Select your fruits and vegetables according to their color

COLOR	MAIN PRODUCTS
Purple	Beets Black currants Blackberries Cranberries Eggplant Grapes Kale Plums Prunes Raspberries Red cabbage Red kidney beans
Green	Broccoli Brussels sprouts Cabbage Cauliflower Chinese cabbage Kale Rutabaga Watercress

Green-yellow	Avocadoes Corn Garden peas Honeydew melons Kiwi Romaine lettuce Spinach Turnips
Orange	Apricots Carrots Mangoes Pumpkins Squash
Orange-yellow	Clementines Grapefruit Lemons Mandarin oranges Melons Nectarines Oranges Papaya Peaches Pears Pineapples Yellow grapes Yellow peppers
Red	Cherries Guava Pink grapefruit Red apples Red onions Strawberries Tomatoes Tomato juice Tomato sauce Watermelons
White and cream	Chicory Garlic Onions Radishes Soy (tofu)

• Eat your fruits and vegetables at the right time of day

1. **In the morning:** eat orange-yellow and orange products, fruit, and fruit juices.

2. **At lunchtime:** you can eat red and white foods, which you can also have with your other meals.

3. **In the evening:** avoid purple foods and eat green foods.

• Your anticancer nutrients

A RANGE OF PROMISING, NATURAL, CHEMOPREVENTIVE COMPOUNDS: THEIR SOURCES, MECHANISMS OF ACTION, AND THE CANCERS THEY ACT ON[1]

ACTIVE SUBSTANCE	NATURAL SOURCE	MECHANISM OF ACTION	ACTS ON CANCER OF THE . . .
Betulinic acid	Widely present in vegetal sources, the best being *Betula* species (birch tree), *Ziziphus* species, *Syzigium* species, *Diospyros* species, and *Paeonia* species	Anti-inflammation, apoptosis, immunomodulation	Skin, ovary, colon, brain, renal cell carcinoma, womb, prostate, leukemia, lung, breast, head and neck
Ellagic acid	Pomegranate juice and pomegranate seed oil, various nuts, blueberried honeysuckle (*Lonicera caerulea*), strawberries and other berries, Arjuna bark (*Terminalia arjuna*), *T. bellerica* leaves and *T. muelleri* bark, leaves, and fruit	Antioxidant, anti-proliferation, anti-inflammation	Skin, pancreas, breast, prostate, colon, intestines, esophagus, bladder, mouth, liver, leukemia, neuroblastoma
Genistein	Soy beans and soy products, red clover (*Trifolium pratense*), Sicilian pistachio (*Pistachi vera*)	Antioxidant, anti-proliferation, anti-angiogenic, anti-inflammation	Prostate, breast, skin, colon, stomach, liver, ovary, pancreas, esophagus, head and neck

Ginkgolide B	*Ginkgo biloba*	Antioxidant, anti-angiogenic	Ovary, breast, brain
Green tea (poly-phenols, EGCG)	Green tea (*Camellia sinensis*)	Antioxidant, anti-mu-tagenic, anti-prolifera-tion, anti-inflammation, anti-angiogenic, immunomodulation	Skin, lung, oral cavity, head and neck, esophagus, stomach, liver, pancreas, small intestine, colon, bladder, prostate, mammary gland
Lupeol	Mangoes, olives, figs, strawberries, red grapes	Antioxidant, anti-mu-tagenic, anti-inflamma-tion, anti-proliferation	Skin, lung, leukemia, pancreas, prostate, colon, liver, head and neck
Luteolin	Artichokes, broccoli, celery, cabbage, spin-ach, green peppers, pomegranate leaves, peppermint, tamarind, cauliflower	Anti-inflammation, anti-allergy, anti-prolif-eration, antioxidant	Ovary, stomach, liver, colon, breast, mouth, prostate, lung, naso-pharynx, cervix, leu-kemia, skin, pancreas, adenocarcinoma of the esophagus
Lycopene	Tomatoes, guava, rosehip, watermelons, papaya, apricots, pink grapefruit; especially plentiful in red toma-toes and tomato-based products	Antioxidant, anti-proliferation, anti-angiogenic, anti-inflammation, immunomodulation	Prostate, lung, breast, stomach, liver, pan-creas, colorectal cancer, head and neck, skin
Pomegranate	Pomegranate, pomegranate juice, pomegranate seeds, pomegranate seed oil (*Punicagranatum*)	Antioxidant, anti-proliferation, anti-angiogenic, anti-inflammation	Prostate, skin, breast, lung, colon, mouth, leukemia
Resveratrol	Red wine, grapes (espe-cially the skin), black-berry bush, peanuts, vines, pine trees	Antioxidant anti-proliferation, anti-angiogenic, anti-inflammation	Ovary, breast, prostate, liver, womb, leukemia, lung, stomach
Turmeric	Turmeric powder (*Curcuma longa*)	Antioxidant, anti-prolif-eration, anti-inflamma-tion, anti-angiogenic, immunomodulation	Skin, lung, oral cavity, head and neck, esoph-agus, stomach, liver, pancreas, small intes-tine, colon, bladder, prostate, mammary gland, lymphoma, soft palate, cervix

• Advice for every profile

If you're a premenopausal woman:

1. Make sure you eat plenty of dairy products and consider taking calcium supplements.

2. Focus on white and green fruits and vegetables, and eat high-fiber foods.

3. If your periods are heavy, eat red meat, lentils, beans, tofu, chick-peas, figs, and apricots.

4. Boost your iron absorption by taking vitamin C supplements.

5. Don't overdo orange fruits and vegetables, especially if you smoke.

6. Make sure you drink plenty of pomegranate juice.

• Calcium content per portion for various dairy products

	PORTION	CALCIUM CONTENT	HOW MUCH YOU'D HAVE TO EAT OR DRINK TO EXCEED 2 G (.1 OZ.) OF CALCIUM A DAY
Camembert	30 g (1.0 oz.)	456	150 g (5.3 oz.)
Cheese spread	30 g (1.0 oz.)	346	180 g (6.3 oz.)
Cow's milk, semi-skimmed, 1 glass of UHT	125 mL (4.4 oz.)	115	18 glasses, i.e, 2.3 L (2.4 qt.)
Emmental	30 g (1.0 oz.)	1,055	60 g (2.1 oz.)
Buttermilk	125 g (4.4 oz.)	97.3	2.5 kg (5.5 lb.)
Fromage blanc, 20% fat	100 g (3.5 oz.)	123	1.5 kg (3.3 lb.)
Goat's milk, whole	1 glass of 125 mL (4.4 oz.)	120	17 glasses, i.e., 2.2 L (2.3 qt.)
Roquefort	30 g (1.0 oz.)	608	100 g (3.5 oz.)
Sheep's milk, whole	1 glass of 125 mL (4.4 oz.)	188	11 glasses, i.e., 1.3 L (1.4 qt.)
Whole-milk natural yogurt	125 g (4.4 oz.)	126	2 kg (4.4 lb.)

If you're a postmenopausal woman:

1. Focus on foods high in calcium and selenium.
2. Don't forget to eat plenty of high-fiber foods.
3. Eat lots of fruits and vegetables, especially green, white, and dark ones.
4. Keep a careful eye on your fat intake.
5. Quercetin is good for you (capers, cocoa, lovage, hot chili peppers).
6. Drink green tea.
7. Drink pomegranate juice.

If you're a man:

1. Avoid beta-carotene, especially in food supplements.
2. Also avoid all multivitamin tablets containing retinol.
3. Limit your vitamin E intake.
4. Don't have too much calcium, so don't eat too much cheese!
5. Eat white (garlic, onions, spring onions, shallots) and red (tomatoes) fruit and vegetables as much as possible. Drink pomegranate juice.
6. Try taking selenium, which is very good for you too, as is quercetin.

• Be physically active, do sport, try *ecologyms*

Incorporate as much walking and physical activity and exertion as you can into your daily routine, or choose some more focused activities.

1. **Aqua aerobics.** Exercising in the water is very effective and particularly recommended if you're overweight. It's also excellent for the joints.
2. **Hiking.** Walking with a group of people in a natural environment is an excellent way of taking moderate exercise without even being aware of it.
3. **Stretching.** This is ideal if you suffer from muscle tension and if you need to relax.

4. **Pilates.** This is an excellent method for strengthening your deep muscles and regaining balance and alignment in your body.

5. **Tai Chi and Qigong.** By focusing on fluidity, balance, and concentration, accompanied by deep breathing, these Far Eastern disciplines are very relaxing.

6. **Power yoga.** This very physical type of yoga gets rid of all psychological and physical stress.